T0234912

Interpretation of semen analysis results

Practical and concise, *Interpretation of semen analysis results: a practical guide* provides a step-by-step approach to every aspect of the interpretation of semen analysis results. While other books focus on basic semen analysis protocol and techniques, few books then go on to actually interpret these results, and provide useful guidance on the significance of different results for infertility assessment. Actual interpretation is greatly facilitated in this guide by a systematic, hands-on approach to identification of the ranges of abnormality that contribute to subfertility in the male. This guide also defines basic concepts, provides clinically essential reference values, and elucidates the often subtle relationships between many sperm characteristics. Once conclusions are reached, the guide offers recommendations for appropriate referral and additional options. Inclusion of vignettes from a wide range of real-life case reports based on a wealth of the author's own experiences helps to illustrate key points. This practical guide is an invaluable resource for all clinicians, scientists and laboratory professionals working with infertile patients.

Interpretation of semen analysis results

A practical guide

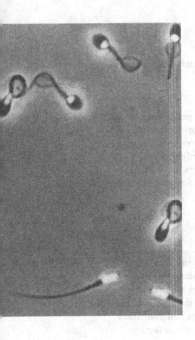

Rajasingam S. Jeyendran

Northwestern University Medical School, Chicago, IL, USA

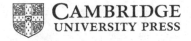

CAMBRIDGE
UNIVERSITY PRESS

CAMBRIDGE UNIVERSITY PRESS
Cambridge, New York, Melbourne, Madrid, Cape Town, Singapore,
São Paulo, Delhi, Dubai, Tokyo, Mexico City

Cambridge University Press
The Edinburgh Building, Cambridge CB2 8RU, UK

Published in the United States of America by Cambridge University Press, New York

www.cambridge.org
Information on this title: www.cambridge.org/9780521799577

First published 2000

A catalogue record for this publication is available from the British Library

ISBN 978-0-521-79957-7 Paperback

Cambridge University Press has no responsibility for the persistence or
accuracy of URLs for external or third-party internet websites referred to in
this publication, and does not guarantee that any content on such websites is,
or will remain, accurate or appropriate. Information regarding prices, travel
timetables, and other factual information given in this work are correct at
the time of first printing but Cambridge University Press does not guarantee
the accuracy of such information thereafter.

Contents

Preface

Infertility plagues one out of eight couples of reproductive age in the United States. Estimates suggest that a significant percentage of such cases result from defective semen quality in the male. Overall, medical and reproductive history of the male spouse notwithstanding, semen analysis remains a major, if not the most important, element of fertility evaluation and therapy.

Male infertility diagnosis throughout the United States is currently practiced by many reproductive endocrinologists, gynecologists, urologists and a significant number of internists and family practitioners. Although many books and publications attempt to facilitate this process through a description of semen analysis methods, none provides an interpretation of semen analysis results. Such interpretative analysis will enable a professional not only to ascertain potential spermatozoon fertilizing capacity, but, should a problem exist, diagnose the exact etiology.

Interpretative semen analysis can thereby identify and often help correct the causes of male factor infertility. By eliminating or minimizing male factor infertility causes, the couple's infertility may be resolved without exposing spouses to the discomforts of hormone therapy and even surgery. Through proficient male fertility analysis, a majority of male reproductive problems may be properly diagnosed and even resolved before resorting to costly medical or surgical interventions. Intracytoplasmic sperm injection utilized in the in vitro fertilization procedure can be another cause for concern: Conducted without a definitive etiologic diagnosis, such a technique can lead to the transmission of genetic mutations to all male offsprings resulting from the procedure. Consequently, an effective and rigorous interpretative approach to semen analysis can greatly facilitate the therapy and reduce the potential risk of the infertile couple and their offspring.

Introduction

Male infertility has been estimated as the primary or contributory factor in more than 40% of infertile couples. Ejaculate analysis is a major tool in male fertility evaluation. Female fertility analysis, being a relatively expensive and complicated process, makes early semen analysis diagnostically appealing. In addition, semen analyses are routinely performed before and/or after cryopreservation, assisted reproductive techniques – such as intrauterine insemination (IUI) and in vitro fertilization (IVF) – vasectomy, vasovasostomy, and for the detection of toxicant exposure to the male reproductive tract.

Over the last few decades, the in-depth study of reproductive function has resulted in many specialties and subspecialties, particularly in andrology. If sperm are freely present in the ejaculate, these specialties help process the sperm for insemination, IVF or intracytoplasmic sperm injection (ICSI). Other subspecialties aspirate the sperm from the reproductive tract (TESE – testicular sperm extraction; MESA: microepididymal sperm aspiration) for ICSI. Rather than conduct an interpretation of semen analysis and thereby correct any problems that might be identified, or first perform fertility enhancing procedures to the ejaculate, many specialists simply refer their patients directly to IVF or ICSI procedure. Although more than 300 laboratories in the United States perform IVF, they remain insufficient to handle every case of male infertility.

Male fertility is dependent upon sperm quantity and quality. Ideally, the fertilizing capacity may be directly appraised by sperm incubation with oocytes under natural reproductive or controlled laboratory conditions. Unfortunately, such a procedure is difficult, if not impossible, for routine semen analysis evaluations.

1

As a practical and viable substitute, several sperm assays have been developed to indirectly infer sperm fertilizing capacity. Standard attributes routinely reported during such diagnostic evaluation include sperm concentration, percent sperm motility, and percent normal sperm morphology. Since large variations may occur even between consecutive ejaculates from the same individual, the fertility potential of the individual under evaluation remains problematic. For example, sperm concentration between ejaculates sampled from the same patient can vary as much as two to threefold, or more. Consequently, only if one or many attributes exhibit extremely poor values can a given result prove deterministic. The interpretation of semen analysis results, therefore, inevitably plays a vital role in the treatment of infertile couples.

The goal of interpretative semen analysis is the quantitative evaluation of spermatozoon fertility potential. However, the presence of non-viable sperm and other agents can interfere with the fertilization process. A determination of such abnormal factors becomes critical for a true interpretation.

Equally baffling, many women will conceive with little or no problem even if their partners display such unusual or 'abnormal' sperm parameters. Semen analysis interpretation as a deterministic evaluation of potential fertility is consequently difficult, and often extremely confusing. Additional tests, such as sperm function evaluations, therefore prove important for the accurate determination of sperm fertility potential.

Sperm function tests provide a reasonable but an indirect gauge of sperm fertility. After all, in vivo conditions prescribe an environment where fertility is contingent on sperm motility and morphology. Sperm able to penetrate and migrate through the cervical mucus are most likely the ones to reach the ampullae of the fallopian tubes and potentially fertilize the oocyte. However, besides inherent sperm qualities that allow sperm to reach the fertilization site, the sperm must be subjected to strict physiological modifications experienced during transit through the internal female organs (capacitation and acrosome reaction). Equally vital is sperm membrane functional integrity, which is a prerequisite for sperm capacitation and the acrosome reaction. Sperm–oocyte contact is impossible without sperm negotiation through the cumulus oophorus and corona radiata, culminating in final penetration of the zona pellucida by acrosome-reacted spermatozoa and fusion of the sperm head with the oocyte vitelline membrane. Once fusion has been satisfactorily achieved, the sperm nucleus must decondense, and male and female chromatin materials fuse to form a full complement of chromosomes.

Interpretative semen analysis is made relatively straightforward with the help of this practical guide. In conjunction with an appropriate companion text, such as the *WHO Laboratory Manual for the Examination of Human Semen and Sperm–Cervical Mucus Interaction* (1999), this guide can greatly facilitate the interpretative process. Other resources on semen analysis include previous publications by the author (Zaneveld & Jeyendran, 1992; Zaneveld et al., 1996; Jeyendran, 1998) and other texts cited at the end of the book (Keel & Webster, 1990; Rowe et al., 1993; Insler & Lunenfeld, 1993; Mortimer, 1994; *Handbook of Andrology*, 1998).

The interpretative analysis elaborated in this text should be used as a constructive guideline. Since even reference values can vary significantly from one publication to the next, accurate interpretation is vital for a consistent and reliable overall diagnosis. Clinicians should utilize this interpretative semen analysis, in conjunction with knowledge of the female partner's fertility status, to make their final recommendation.

Hypotheses on fertile ejaculate identification

The primary purpose of semen analysis is the determination of spermatozoon fertility potential. Such interpretation and fertility potential determination involve different conceptual frameworks. To enhance overall understanding of interpretative procedure and its interrelationship with sperm fertility potential, consider the following conceptual outline:

Although the fertilization process is fairly well understood, existing scientific knowledge provides few specific parameters regarding the fertilizing capacity of any particular ejaculate. Granted, an infertile ejaculate can be identified with some facility and certainty when one sperm parameter is significantly or absolutely abnormal. Realistically, the spermatozoon is an extremely complex cell that becomes infertile when any one of a number of highly sensitive biochemical, physiological or morphologic entities is disturbed. Such complexity makes fertilization evaluation even more difficult when one or several of these attributes deviate only slightly from the statistical mean.

The goal of semen analysis, ultimately, is to evaluate whether an ejaculate is potentially fertile or not. Conducting a large battery of assays will ensure some degree of certainty. Unfortunately, the interpretative challenge then becomes which of the many available assays should be performed.

A single test assay capable of identifying several different sperm attributes would be ideal. In fact, such assays are available, mainly as sperm processing procedures for IUI and other assisted reproductive technologies. For example, any routine sperm selection technique such as the Swim-Up Method, washing through density gradients (colloidal suspension of silica particles, Nycodenz), or adherence column filtration methods (glass wool or Sephadex) yields a sperm subpopulation with significantly higher quality. The sperm obtained as a result of utilizing these techniques generally improves several sperm attributes to the point of reaching (or satisfying) reference value criteria for different sperm variables. Further research and development on these unconventional fertility evaluation procedures are needed either to standardize and establish routine sperm test assays, or to improve or abandon them when experience renders them useless.

To complicate matters further, a majority of sperm in any given ejaculate cannot be absolutely classified as either normal or abnormal. Sperm morphology can vary from virtually flawless to unequivocally abnormal, with a broad range in-between. Similarly, 'normal' sperm motility has differing motion characteristics, including various degrees of functional forward progression. The acrosome reaction can be induced with different agents via different mechanisms to different effect. Other sperm attributes exhibit equally broad gradients between 'normal' and 'abnormal' accepted norms. Consequently, different grades of potential fertility can exist within the same ejaculate sample, further contributing to the ambiguity of the designations 'fertile' and 'infertile.' In place of 'normalcy,' therefore, reference values have been prescribed by the *WHO Laboratory Manual* (1999) to facilitate standardization and analysis.

Consider: An ejaculate, after fractionation by glass wool column filtration, had an initial aliquot sperm population with significantly higher motility, functional membrane integrity, acrosin content, and higher hamster oocytes penetration potential than subsequent fractions or the original ejaculate. Such evidence suggests that, given a sperm population of specified normalcy, a subpopulation is extractable which can deliver even higher fertility potential (display ranges well above prescribed reference values). An assay which facilitates such optimal segregation of particularly fertile spermatozoa from any given ejaculate would greatly aid in the overall evaluation and interpretation of the semen analysis.

Subfertile or non-fertile (sterile) sperm present within the ejaculate compromise the fertility potential of fertile sperm. Under in vivo conditions the cervical mucus operates as a biological filter, preventing the entry of most abnormal, non-motile, and non-viable sperm into the upper female reproductive tract.

Within the laboratory, a penetration assay using glass wool filtered sperm was compromised by addition of killed sperm and sperm retained in the filter. The overall fertile sperm competency was somewhat jeopardized by inferior sperm in the same ejaculate. Clearly, if we accept that the presence of dead or infertile sperm compromises the overall fertility potential of the ejaculate; these poor quality elements must also be assessed.

Note: Even if an ejaculate is initially diagnosed infertile, the removal of subfertile or non-fertile sperm could, in fact, render the remaining sperm fertile and useful for reproductive techniques, such as IUI and IVF. Therefore, dismissing an ejaculate as 'infertile' outright before attempting these additional procedures is premature and potentially wasteful.

Male reproductive system background

In an effort to provide background for the interpretative evaluation of semen analysis results, a brief description of the male reproductive system is provided. This should refresh the reader's basic knowledge, and provide a basic anatomical and physiological framework. The overview includes functional anatomy, endocrinology, emission and ejaculation, spermatozoa description, sexual stimulation, and semen collection.

Functional anatomy

The male sexual anatomy can arbitrarily be divided into four parts:

- The testis: male gonads producing the spermatozoa
- The epididymis and vas deferens: organs that mature, store, and transport spermatozoa
- The accessory sex glands: organs that supply most of the fluid portions (or seminal plasma) of the semen at ejaculation
- The penis: organ for the delivery of semen

The testis: male gonads producing the spermatozoa
The testicles are a pair of reproductive glands located outside the body within a skin pouch, the scrotum. They are each oval-shaped and approximately 25 milliliters in volume. They are designed to fulfil a double function: the production of sexual hormone, directly interrelated to its second function, the production of spermatozoa (spermatogenesis). Within the limits set by the flexible but unstretchable albuginea, the testis is composed of

a large number of lobules. Each lobule consists of a large number of tubules (seminiferous tubules) all connected to the hilus and a marginal rete testis where the sperm are generated. The seminiferous tubules are surrounded by a basement membrane. Within the tubules, two types of cells are found: the ever-multiplying germ cells that ultimately result in the formation of spermatozoa, and Sertoli cells that provide the biochemical milieu for the support of the evolving germ cells in their intricate metamorphosis from spermatocyte, to spermatid, and finally to spermatozoon. Besides, the lobules also consist of cell clusters in the intertubular spaces (interstitial or Leydig cells) that constitute the endocrine part of the gonad. The interstitial tissue consists of collagenous fibers, blood and lymph vessels, and various types of connective cells.

Spermatogenesis is an elaborate cell differentiation process, starting with the germ cell (spermatogonia) and terminating with a fully differentiated highly specialized cell called the spermatozoon. The spermatogonia is located at the base of the seminiferous epithelium, and consists of two classes: Type A and Type B. In the human, the most basic Type A spermatogonia are the pale type (Ap) and dark type (Ad). Ap spermatogonia divide mitotically into Ap spermatogonia and Type B spermatogonia. The Ap spermatogonia remain attached to the basal membrane and continually replenish themselves. Therefore, spermatogenesis can continue until old age. The Ad spermatogonia rarely divide and are tentatively considered as dormant reserve germ cells.

Type B spermatogonia derive from Ap spermatogonia and divide mitotically to produce primary spermatocytes. The primary spermatocytes undergo two meiotic divisions: the first division gives rise to two pseudo-diploid secondary spermatocytes. The second division, in turn, gives rise to four haploid (23 chromosomes) spermatids, two of which carry the X (maternal) chromosome and two the Y (paternal) chromosome. These spermatids subsequently undergo metamorphosis and develop into spermatozoa through various morphological changes, referred to as spermiogenesis. They are then released into the seminiferous tubule. Spermatogenesis requires approximately 70 days in humans.

Sperm production is constant and continues throughout the adult life of the human male. Sperm not ejaculated gradually die and dissolve (cytolysis) like any other cells in the body.

The epididymis, and vas deferens: organs that mature, store, and transport spermatozoa

Spermatozoa leave the testis by way of the rete testis, and a number of vasa (ductuli) efferentia. These ductuli join to form a single and very long, highly convoluted duct that comprises the tubular portion of the epididymis, a structure only a few centimeters long. The head (caput) of the epididymis attaches to the testicle. The tail (cauda) leads into the vas deferens, a muscular tube of approximately 37 centimeters that extends from the epididymis and testis in the scrotum, and enters the body through the inguinal canal to reach the urethra. At its urethral end, the vas enlarges into an ampullary portion, forms the ejaculatory ducts with the excretory canals of the seminal vesicles, and joins the urethra.

Full spermatozoon maturation and fertilizing ability cannot be achieved until passage through the epididymis is realized. During this passage, the spermatozoa also attain the capacity to be motile, although they ordinarily do not move under their own control until after ejaculation. Epididymal passage of spermatozoa requires from 4 to 10 days.

Spermatozoa remain motionless in the male genital tract, their transport primarily accomplished by fluid flow in the testis and, thereafter, by organ contractions. The site of sperm storage is primarily the tail (cauda) of the epididymis but also the vas deferens. Few spermatozoa find their way into the seminal vesicles and degenerate. These sperm are generally found in the terminal portion of the ejaculate.

The accessory sex glands: organs that supply most of the fluid portion (or seminal plasma) of the semen at ejaculation

Humans possesses three accessory sex glands: the seminal vesicles, prostate gland, and Cowper's gland (bulbourethral gland). The fluids from these glands provide the vehicle for spermatozoa transport and sustenance, and are collectively called the seminal plasma of the ejaculate. The seminal vesicles enter the vas deferens at its ampullary portion and produce, for instance, the fructose and coagulating proteins present in seminal plasma. The prostate gland is located at the junction of the vas and the urethra. Its fluid is characterized by the presence of zinc, citric acid, and acid phosphatase, producing the typical odor of semen. The prostate also secretes the enzyme(s) that liquefies the semen coagulum. The Cowper's glands are situated immediately distal to the prostate gland and empty into the bulbous urethra. The fluids from this gland are thought to wet the urethra prior to ejaculation.

The penis: organ for the delivery of semen

Penile erection is required for penetration into the vagina for semen deposition. The human penis erects by means of vascular engorgement. Briefly, engorgement results from peripheral vasodilatation brought about by parasympathetic impulses passed via the pelvic nervi erigentes. The nervus erigens emerges bilaterally from the spinal cord at the level of sacral segments 2 and 3 and pass primarily via the pelvic plexus and finally into the arterial walls.

The penile arteries, derived from the internal pudendal artery, are coiled in the corpus cavernosum penis. During erection, these arteries straighten out and fill the sinuses (cavernous sinuses) of the erectile tissues with blood. The penile vasculature does not include a typical capillary system, so blood is emptied directly into the cavernous sinuses. This increases pressure within the penis and in turn compresses the thin-walled veins lying in the tunica albuginea. The penis then becomes engorged with blood, enlarges and stiffens.

During erection, the glans penis becomes especially prominent and turgid because it not only receives blood from the dorsal and deep penile arteries, but also from the bulb artery via the corpus spongiosum, an extension.

Testicular endocrine control

The hormonal regulation of testis begins in the hypothalamus, which synthesizes and releases, in a pulsatile manner, a decapeptide gonadotropin-releasing hormone (GnRH). This hormone regulates the secretion of pituitary hormones, which in turn, through a complex feedback mechanism between the various hormones, regulate testicular hormone secretion.

Two pituitary gonadotropic hormones are present in the male: luteinizing hormone (LH) and follicle-stimulating hormone (FSH). These glycoprotein hormones are identical to the gonadotropins of the female. LH stimulates the Leydig cells to convert cholesterol to testosterone. FSH induces the Sertoli cells to form androgen binding protein, which may assist testosterone movement toward the seminiferous tubular lumen and the epididymis. FSH also induces the Sertoli cells to convert testosterone to 5-dihydrotestosterone (5α-DHT), 17β-estradiol, and also to produce inhibin. The 5α-DHT is more active than testosterone, and along with 17β-estradiol, is involved in the development and function of the accessory sex glands, penis, scrotum, the secondary male sex characteristics, libido and potency. Testosterone is responsible for the maintenance of spermatogenesis, whereas FSH is needed to initiate spermatogenesis at the onset of puberty.

Hormonal integration of the hypothalamic–pituitary–testicular axis is a basic requirement for normal spermatogenesis, and any hormonal imbalance may result in the partial or complete compromise of fertility potential.

For example, if the normal testosterone route is blocked due to a defect in the androgen receptor protein, then spermatogenesis is fundamentally compromised. Such a condition results in testicular feminization and is known as androgen insensitivity syndrome. Another condition involves the absence of 5α-DHT, caused by enzyme 5α-reductase deficiency, also resulting in testicular feminization. The patient will have clinical symptoms other than the overt compromise of fertility potential, which can greatly aid in the diagnosis.

Emission and ejaculation

The male sexual response consists of four distinct stages: Erection, emission, ejaculation and detumescence. Emission and ejaculation are two components responsible for the deposition and expulsion of semen, respectively.

Emission begins as coordinated sequential contractions originating in the testis efferent ducts, the epididymis tail, and the convoluted portion of vas deferens. Contractions proceed in an integrated manner and propel the sperm into the prostatic urethra.

Prostatic fluid is the first component, followed by the sperm-rich fraction from the ampulla and the vas deferens. Finally, the seminal vesicular fluid is deposited into the prostatic urethra. During emission, the bladder neck and external urethral sphincter are closed to contain the deposited seminal fluid. Physical closure of the bladder neck is essential for the prevention of retrograde semen flow back into the bladder.

The initial emission phase is followed by ejaculation. Ejaculation may be defined as the actual discharge of semen from the penis. The ejaculatory event consists of external sphincter relaxation, followed by rhythmic prostate contractions. Bulbospongiosus muscles then propel the semen in an antigrade manner out of the external urethral meatus.

The emission process is mediated by the sympathetic nervous system via adrenergic mechanisms, arising in the spinal cord at the thoracic 10 to lumbar 2 vertebra level. The pathways for these efferent neural signals originate from the lumbar 1 paravertebral ganglion.

Ejaculation, in contrast, is mediated by both parasympathetic (sacral vertebra 2–4) and somatic nervous systems via the pudendal nerve. The neural efferent signal for ejaculation originates in the spinal cord at the sacral vertebra 2–4 level and travels via a somatic pathway along the pudendal nerve motor division.

Ejaculation normally occurs in a definite sequence. First, a small amount of Cowper's gland fluid is extruded. Next, the prostatic fluid and sperm-rich fraction from the ampulla and the vas deferens (averaging approximately 0.5 milliliter) is released. Finally the secretions of the seminal vesicles (averaging approximately 1.5–3.0 milliliters) is released. The three portions become mixed and the seminal coagulum is formed. This gel normally spontaneously liquefies in about 20 minutes. Within this thick gel matrix, the trapped spermatozoa are immotile, until becoming active following liquefaction.

Sexual stimulation

The sexual stimulatory signals are modulated by inhibitory and excitatory stimuli from higher brain centers. These centers include the anterior thalamic, preoptic, hypothalamic, and forebrain nuclei. Semen quality and quantity therefore at least partially depend on higher brain excitement levels.

In animal husbandry, bulls are teased by allowing them to mount a cow or a dummy a few times prior to ejaculate collection. Such continued higher brain stimulation increases the overall quality and quantity of ejaculate obtained. Similarly in humans, studies have demonstrated that seminal pouch collection during actual coitus yields better ejaculate than that obtained through masturbation alone.

Semen collection

Masturbation is the most recommended collection method. Non-recommended methods include coitus interruptus (withdrawal), where the loss of initial semen fraction and vaginal fluid contamination are possible. For similar reasons, oral semen collection and vaginal drainage collection is not recommended. For men concerned with religious or other personal contingencies and therefore unwilling to masturbate, the seminal pouch collection method can be recommended.

Impotence due to psychosomatic or medical reasons (such as diabetes or spinal cord injuries) may require vibratory or electro-stimulation techniques. During electro-stimulation, a portion of the ejaculate flows back into the bladder. Catheterization of the bladder is therefore required to obtain all of the ejaculated spermatozoa. In addition, use of Viagra or similar prescription drugs may be useful in correcting semen collection problems due to impotence.

Several ejaculates from the same subject need to be analyzed to obtain objective data. Optimally, ejaculates should be analyzed every 2 to 3 weeks until four ejaculates have been studied. For convenience, at least two ejaculates should be analyzed 1 month apart. If either one of these two ejaculates shows abnormalities, additional ejaculates should then be studied to better assess the clinical diagnosis.

Intersample variation is mostly attributable to duration of sexual abstinence between samples. A semen specimen should therefore be collected by masturbation after the standard sexual abstinence period recommended for semen analysis of 2 to 3 days. Another semen sample should be collected after a sexual abstinence period corresponding to the couple's usual coital frequency, thereby obtaining a more realistic assessment of typical semen quality for that couple.

Semen quality varies over time. All fertility patients need to monitor their semen quality at least once or twice a year, during the duration of treatment.

Careful instructions must be given to the patient before ejaculate production. The collection method and subsequent handling of the ejaculate prior to the analysis must be fully acknowledged and understood, particularly if abnormalities are subsequently discovered.

Preferably the specimen should be collected at the laboratory or delivered to the laboratory within 20 minutes of production, and definitely within 1 hour. The specimen should be protected from temperature extremes during transit and delivery. To maintain proper temperature when the weather is cold, for example, the specimen should be kept close to the body (body temperature, e.g., in the inside pocket of a jacket) during transportation to the laboratory. Ideally, samples should be collected and analyzed in the laboratory.

Spermatozoon anatomy and physiology

The typical spermatozoon is about 50 μm long and consists of a head and tail. The head is oval and flat in shape, tapering apically, measuring 4.0–5.0 μm in length, 2.5–3.5 μm in width and the length to width ratio of 1.50 to 1.75. The sperm nucleus comprises approximately 65% of the head and consists of tightly packed chromosomal material (largely DNA) and basic protein. The anterior portion of the head is covered by a sac-like structure called the acrosome (galea capitis, head cap) that contains enzymes essential for the sperm progression through the different layers of cells surrounding the egg and its zona pellucida.

The tail is about ten times the length of the head. The tail is enclosed within a thin sheath and possesses two central fibers within nine outer pairs of fibers that start at the neck and run to the tip of the tail. The midpiece is the anterior portion of the tail and consists of a sheath surrounding tightly packed mitochondria. The junction between tailpiece and midpiece is marked by the presence of a ring called the annulus. Collectively, the fibers, powered by mitochondria in the midpiece, are called the axial filament complex, which is the main organ for sperm motility.

As the spermatozoa develop in the testis, the spermatid cell wall collapses around the sperm, forming the outermost plasma membrane and the cytoplasmic droplet which contains part of the excess cytoplasm of the spermatid cell. This droplet is originally located at the neck of the spermatozoon but moves down to the posterior portion of the midpiece as the sperm matures in the epididymis. The cytoplasmic droplet is released during ejaculation if the spermatozoon has sufficiently matured.

Spermatozoon motility is the single most important factor in sperm transport through the cervix, although other factors play a role. At mid-cycle, at the peak of cervical mucus quality, spermatozoa not trapped in the coagulum enter the cervix almost instantly (within 30–60 seconds of ejaculation). Some spermatozoa migrate and are transported into the uterus and tubes rapidly. Others are stored in cervical mucus and released continually for 2 to 4 days. Observation of the sperm in the cervical mucus 7 days postcoital is not uncommon.

Of the millions of spermatozoa normally ejaculated into the vagina, only 0.1–1% reach the uterus. Of these, merely 1000–5000 spermatozoa can actually be found in the fallopian tube ampulla, i.e., at the site of fertilization. All excess spermatozoa are removed through phagocytosis by leukocytes that enter the uterus in large numbers approximately 10 to 24 hours after first spermatozoon entry. Spermatozoa may also leave the genital tract by passing into the peritoneal cavity via the fimbriated end of the fallopian tube. Spermatozoa have been found in the fallopian tube ampulla up to 85 hours after coitus.

To be transported to and through the tubes, the sperm must remain, by their own motility in suspension, within the female internal reproductive organs secreted fluids. Sperm motility is also needed to avoid being phagocytized by polymorphous white blood cells contained in the body fluids.

In addition, spermatozoa are also transported through the uterus and fallopian tubes by movement of cilia present on the luminal surface of the endometrial cells and by the contractions of the female genital tract.

The first spermatozoa reach the ampullary portion of the fallopian tubes within 5 to 15 minutes following insemination. Standard migration time for the majority of the spermatozoa reaching the fertilization site is 2 to 24 hours after coitus; however, the spermatozoa, even though fully mature, cannot fertilize an oocyte until certain biochemical and morphological changes take place. Spermatozoa normally undergo these changes (called 'capacitation') in the cervix, uterine cavity and the fallopian tubes during the estrogenic phase.

Sperm–oocyte interaction

Spermatozoa are biochemically altered during capacitation. A number of changes occur in sperm head membrane and structures. Certain surface agents are removed that would otherwise prevent spermatozoon penetration through the layers surrounding the egg. Capacitation permits the 'acrosome reaction' to occur as the spermatozoon comes into contact with the egg. The acrosome reaction involves the fusion of the plasma membrane with the outer acrosomal membrane, their subsequent vesiculation, and finally their disappearance. The inner acrosomal membrane is thereby exposed, aiding in laying a path for the spermatozoon to penetrate through the zona pellucida.

Fertilization takes place in the ampulla of the fallopian tube. Observers contend the human oocyte (egg) remains maximally fertile for 12 to 24 hours after ovulation. When the spermatozoon reaches the oocyte, the egg is surrounded by three layers. From the outside inward, these are the cumulus oophorus, the corona radiata, and the zona pellucida. The fertilizing spermatozoon rapidly penetrates these layers, leaving them apparently intact. Only spermatozoa from the same species as the egg can penetrate the zona, an immunological, species-selective natural protective mechanism. The zona pellucida also provides a barrier to polyspermy, since only a single spermatozoon is allowed to penetrate.

When the spermatozoon enters the perivitelline space, the cortical reaction is induced and also triggers completion of the second meiotic egg division.

The spermatozoon attaches sideways onto the surface of the vitelline membrane at the postnuclear cap area and fuses with the egg membrane. The sperm tail first disrupts at the midpiece. The fibrous tail sheet and the nine outer dense fibers disperse next, followed finally by the axoneme and head decondensation liberating the male chromatids.

The male pronucleus then begins to develop along the periphery at the ovum entry site. Then the male pronucleus moves toward the egg center where the female pronucleus is located. The nucleoli subsequently disappear, the pronuclear membranes break down, and the chromosomes from each respective pronuclei combine along the equatorial cleavage spindle. The first cleavage follows immediately, thus culminating the fertilization process and restoring diploidy.

Semen analysis interpretation

Semen analysis is usually performed as part of the comprehensive investigation of an infertile couple. Interpretation of these analysis results plays a vital role in the overall treatment of infertile couples. All semen samples, regardless of collection circumstances, have the potential for providing at least some meaningful information, and should therefore be analyzed.

Semen analysis can involve several distinct techniques and procedures. The basic procedure is simply called **routine semen analysis**, composed of:

Macroscopic analysis
Determination of semen appearance, coagulation and liquefaction time, color and odor, viscosity, and volume.

Microscopic analysis
Determination of the presence of non-sperm cellular elements, sperm agglutination, sperm concentration, sperm motility, and sperm morphology.

Standard parameters are routinely used to indicate the potential fertility 'status,' of a specimen, i.e., sperm concentration, motility, and morphology. While important, they have significant limitations, unless these variables are highly abnormal.

A number of highly *specialized semen analyses* have therefore been developed to circumvent this deficiency and aid in a more accurate diagnosis of male factor infertility and its etiology, and include:

(i) *Sperm function tests* that determine the ability of spermatozoa to migrate into the cervical mucus or other adequate substitute.

•

These tests also evaluate the sperm capacity to respond to hypo-osmotic stress or to exclude supravital dyes, to undergo membrane changes (such as sperm capacitation and acrosome reaction). They also determine sperm ability to bind to the human zona pellucida, or the sperm ability to penetrate into zona free hamster oocytes.

(ii) *Sperm nuclear integrity tests* determine the normal chromatin condensation of the nucleus, and ascertain the stability of sperm DNA.

(iii) *Antisperm antibody tests* for the blood serum, seminal plasma, spermatozoa, and cervical mucus.

(iv) *Biochemical analysis of spermatozoa* to determine the activity of fertilization enzymes such as sperm acrosin and metabolic enzymes such as sperm creatine phosphokinase. The analysis also may determine the adenosine triphosphate content as well as reactive oxygen species.

(v) *Chemical analysis of seminal plasma* determines the concentration of zinc, citric acid, acid phosphatase, fructose (reducing sugar) and α-glucosidase content, including seminal plasma pH. Note that one specific chemical marker for each accessory sex gland is sufficient to determine the respective gland's contribution.

Such an assessment reveals spermatozoon testicular output, functional properties of spermatozoa, and accessory sexual glands secretory function.

The following section provides an interpretative description of both routine and specialized semen analysis; where pertinent, individual interpretations are cross-referenced between different parameters to facilitate the overall interpretation.

ROUTINE SEMEN ANALYSIS

Includes both macroscopic and microscopic examination of the ejaculate:

Macroscopic analysis interpretations

Appearance

What is it?
Semen is characteristically turbid.

How is it described?
Ejaculate turbidity can be described as transparent, translucent, or opaque.

Abnormalities?
Large amount of debris or leukocytes may render the specimen opaque.

Significance
Sperm presence in the seminal fluid makes the semen appear turbid and is used as a very rough estimate of semen quality for animals, not for humans. In animal husbandry, semen transparency typically indicates poor sperm quantity, necessitating a repeat collection. In humans, the relationship between semen transparency and quality is ambiguous.

Recommendation
Semen appearance is of no clinical value in the analysis of human ejaculate.

Coagulation and liquefaction

What is it?
Immediately following ejaculation, semen normally coagulates into a gelatinous mass and then liquefies within 20 minutes

when at room temperature, or within 15 to 20 minutes at 37 °C.

How is it determined?

The time required for the gelatinous mass to liquefy.

Abnormalities?

The lack (absence) of coagulation may indicate ejaculatory duct obstruction or the congenital absence of the seminal vesicles (since coagulating proteins originate within the seminal vesicles). If the ejaculate has not liquefied after 120 minutes, the sample is abnormal. Prolonged liquefaction time or complete absence of liquefaction is most likely due to poor prostatic secretion (since the liquefying enzymes are derived from the prostate gland).

Significance

Normal semen may contain many small gel-like clots ('proteinaceous' bodies) or corpuscles which do not liquefy. The significance of these clots is not known. The exact liquefaction time is of no diagnostic importance unless more than two hours elapse without a state change.

Recommendation

For a semen sample that will not liquefy either for semen analysis, artificial insemination or for use in assisted reproductive technology (ART), the ejaculate can be mixed either with an equal amount of semen extender, or forced in and out of a 3-milliliter syringe attached to a 18-gauge needle until the sample becomes more pliable. Specifically, treatment with liquefying agents such as 5% α-amylase, Alevair, or trypsin is possible. The addition of bromelin at 1g per liter, plasmin 0.35–0.50 casein units per milliliter, or chymotrypsin 150 USP per milliliter may also assist in liquefying an ejaculate.

Color and odor

What is it?

The color and smell of semen.

How is it described?

Semen is usually whitish-grey, pearl white or a yellowish opalescent fluid. Semen odor is unmistakable and pungent because of spermine oxidation.

Abnormalities?

Any abnormal color or odor may suggest an inappropriate collection container, and may have nothing to do with actual sperm condition. Should that possibility be ruled out, accurate medical diagnosis becomes vital: jaundice may color the semen yellow. A reddish color is usually due to red blood cells, a condition called hematospermia (See 'Hematospermia,' page 32). Urine contamination of the ejaculate may also change semen color and odor. A yellow tint is probably due to carotene pigment (carotene pigment in semen is associated with higher fertility in the bovine). Drugs such as methylene blue and pyridium may also color semen.

Significance

Semen color and odor have no significance in the evaluation of spermatozoon fertilizing potential.

Recommendation

Should sperm quality be compromised due to an inappropriate collection container, repeating the procedure using a recommended semen collection container and properly supervised collection process is advised.

Viscosity

What is it?

After ejaculation the semen is a non-homogeneous coagulum which becomes more fluid after liquefaction. Viscosity measures the friction between various seminal fluid components as they slide by one another.

How is it measured?

Viscosity in semen may be measured in millimeters by the length of the 'spinnbarkeit,' or the 'threadiness.' Up to 40 mm 'spinnbarkeit' length is considered normal. The coagulum may be absent from semen samples that are highly viscous. Coagulum and viscosity can be differentiated by swirling the vessel, since the coagulum will not conform to the shape of the container. Viscous fluid will conform to its environment, however, albeit slowly.

Viscosity (except when no liquefaction is exhibited) can be appraised subjectively by sticking a wooden stick (like a tooth pick) and observing if a thread is formed.

Abnormalities?

If the 'spinnbarkeit' (or 'threadiness') is longer than 60 mm in length, viscosity is considered abnormal. Abnormality is also considered if no thread at all is formed due to insignificant lique-faction.

Significance

The relationship between viscosity and fertility is unknown. High viscosity, however, combined with poor sperm motility, can lead to a marked decrease in fertilization capacity due to problems with delivery: the poor or total absence of sperm-release into the cervical mucus.

Recommendation

The same agents used to lyse the coagulum artificially, such as α-amylase and Alevair, may be employed before the artificial insemination of a viscous ejaculate. Alternatively, dilution with a semen extender may adequately suffice to reduce ejaculate viscosity.

Volume

What is it?

Volume is measured in milliliters and typically ranges from 2 to 4 milliliters. The volume depends primarily on accessory sexual gland secretions. The seminal vesicle contributes between 1.5 and 5.0 milliliter, the prostate 0.2 to 1.0 milliliter, and a small fraction is contributed from the bulbourethral gland. About 0.2 milliliter containing the actual spermatozoa is derived from the vas deferens, epididymis and testicles.

How is it measured?

Semen volume is measured to the nearest 0.1 milliliter with a graduated pipette, centrifuge tube or syringe.

Abnormalcy?

According to the *WHO Laboratory Manual* (1999), the reference value for semen volume is 2.0 milliliters; however, for clinical purposes, semen volume is differentiated into three useful categories to facilitate interpretation and diagnosis.

- A man is aspermic if he produces no semen at all after orgasm.
- He is hypospermic if less than 0.5 milliliter of semen is ejaculated.
- He is hyperspermic if the ejaculate measures above 6.0 milliliters.

Aspermia may be due to a clinical problem:

- transurethral or open surgical resections of the bladder neck or prostate
- bilateral sympathectomy
- bilateral retroperitoneal lymphadenectomy
- extensive pelvic surgery (particularly proctectomy and colectomy)
- diabetic visceral neuropathy
- antihypertensive drugs that block sympathetic tone
- electro-stimulation to obtain an ejaculate (patients with spinal cord injury).

How is it determined?

Total lack of an ejaculate following orgasm (aspermia) or a very small semen volume (hypospermia) following ejaculation. Any voided urine following masturbation must be evaluated immediately. If spermatozoa are present, then retrograde semen flow back into the bladder has occurred and the condition is referred to as retrograde flow of semen.

WHAT IS RETROGRADE FLOW OF SEMEN?

(erroneously referred to as: 'retrograde ejaculation')

This condition occurs when semen flows backwards into the urinary bladder during orgasm. Such retrograde semen flow can

be caused by any process that interferes with sympathetic inner-
vation or the compromised anatomic integrity of the bladder
neck's smooth muscle (See 'Emission and ejaculation,' page 13).
Typically, the urinary sphincter is closed during ejaculation to
prevent retrograde semen flow into the bladder. But, if the
sphincter is not contracted for whatever reason, the ejaculate
may flow back into the bladder rather than proceed through the
urethra.

SIGNIFICANCE

General practice today suggests that all voided urine should be
collected immediately following masturbation. Often, the
patient is instructed to ingest bicarbonates to alkalinize the
urine. The urine is subsequently centrifuged, and the sperm con-
centrated for analysis or insemination processing. The bladder
can also be catheterized ('washed') with buffered physiological
solution. A few milliliters left in the bladder help to neutralize the
urine effects. Following orgasm, the patient may void or the
bladder is recatheterized for specimen collection. However, urine
in excess of 40% volume-to-volume concentration has deleterious effects on sperm function (even when urine pH and osmolality are neutralized).

RECOMMENDATION

Immediately following orgasm, voided urine should be sequen-
tially collected in approximately 5 milliliter aliquots and checked
for spermatozoa. If spermatozoa are present, then the aliquots
containing the sperm should be mixed immediately with three to
four times media volume and centrifuged at 500 g for 3 minutes.
The resultant sperm pellet should be resuspended in sperm
media and subsequently analyzed for sperm quality or processed
for artificial insemination. Typically, the first aliquot will contain
almost all of the ejaculate. Utilizing this procedure, the deleterious effects of urine can be superseded. To facilitate the recovery
of viable sperm, one may collect the aliquots of urine in buffered
physiological solution.

Hypospermia (volume less than 0.5 milliliter) may be due to procedural causes or clinical factors.

Procedural causes
(i)   incomplete collection (partially missing the jar)
(ii)   spillage following sample collection
(iii) partial ejaculation due to incomplete orgasm (probably brought about by anxiety, stress, disapproval and embarrassment about masturbation, etc.).
(iv)   an insufficient period of sexual abstinence between ejaculations.

Clinical factors
Hypospermia is associated with four different conditions, which include:

(i)   hypospermia without spermatozoa in semen, with pH less than 7.4
(ii)   hypospermia with spermatozoa in semen, with pH less than 7.4
(iii) hypospermia with spermatozoa in semen, with pH more than 7.8
(iv)   hypospermia without (or low numbers of) spermatozoa in semen, with pH more than 7.8.

Condition (i) could be due to ejaculatory duct obstruction or congenital absence of the seminal vesicles. Semen chemistries should be investigated (See 'Chemical analysis of seminal plasma' page 70). Such symptoms are associated with either partial or complete absence of fructose (produced by the seminal vesicles). However, normal zinc and acid phosphatase content with acidic pH (produced by the prostate gland) should be present.

Condition (ii) could be due to obstruction of the seminal vesicular opening by a mucus-like plug, producing high sperm concentration. The obstructing plug may dissolve spontaneously, leading to normal ejaculate volumes; but more often than not the obstacle actually enlarges, causing azoospermia over time. (See 'A Case report: obstruction at the colliculus seminalis,' page 71.) Stricture of the seminal vesicular duct, probably due to inflammation, may also result in this condition.

Condition (iii) could be due to any of the following four situations:

- a partial or incomplete retrograde flow of semen. Post-ejaculated, voided urine must be examined.
- accessory sex gland impairment, for example, that caused by inflammation or cancer (especially if the pH is more than 9.0).
- oxymetholone, thioridazine, phenoxybenzamine and guanethidine treatment.
- addiction to narcotics such as heroin, or methadone.

Condition (iv) could be due to hypoandrogenism leading to impaired spermatogenesis, while some fructose may still be present.

Hyperspermia (volume more than 6.0 milliliters) is due to either:
(i) a long period of sexual abstinence; or
(ii) accessory sex gland fluid overproduction, probably from the seminal vesicle. (In the author's own laboratory experience, the largest volume measured from a single ejaculate was 14.7 milliliters.)

Significance

Overall, semen volume has a minimal effect on spermatozoon fertilizing potential. However, semen volume determination can aid in the identification of abnormal semen etiology by providing a measurable parameter.

Precaution

Typically, patients feel that, in private, they produce more semen than that collected in the laboratory. Patient have been known to ejaculate twice into the same container in order to increase the overall volume for a single sample; others have even voided urine into the receptacle to accomplish this feat.

Recommendation

▶ *For aspermia:* if a consequence of retrograde semen flow, retrieve sperm from the bladder and process for artificial insemination.
▶ *For hypospermia:* artificial insemination may be a solution if the patient has no other problem. Based on diagnosis, refer to a urologist for evaluation and correction or to an assisted reproductive specialist.
▶ *For hyperspermia:* if fertility problems occur, process to concentrate the sperm for artificial insemination.

A drop of semen is placed on a clean microscope slide and covered with a coverslip. Presence of sperm and subjective percent motility and forward progression should be estimated. If only poor or no sperm motility following dilution with a buffered physiological solution is encountered, inappropriately prepared buffered physiological solution or contaminated counting chambers could be causing the artificially decreased sperm motility. In such cases, the media itself should be changed or the counting chamber should be cleaned, and observations repeated.

Non-sperm cellular elements

Cellular elements such as leukocytes, erythrocytes, epithelial cells, fungi, bacteria, and protozoa may be present in the seminal fluid.

Leukocytes

Some leukocytes, possibly originating from the prostate, may be present in the seminal fluid and are typically of no significance. However, large numbers of leukocytes in the ejaculate can become significant, the condition referred to as leukocytospermia.

What is leukocytospermia?

Moderate to heavy amounts (more than five leukocytes per high-power field, or greater than one million per milliliter), of leukocytes present along with seminal debris may suggest a possible accessory sex glands infection. Such infection is likely to affect sperm motility.

Significance

Leukocytes in semen produce oxidative stress (the generation of free oxygen radicals) and cytotoxic cytokines secretions (lymphokines and monokines). These products may interfere with sperm progression. Leukocytes may also be a factor in sperm agglutination. Occasionally, macrophages and polymorphs are visible, phagocytizing spermatozoa.

Staining for leukocytes is advisable when more than five leukocytes are seen per each high-power field. The simplest technique is the ortho-toluidine blue stain for peroxidase-positive cells. The leukocytes stain brown and are quantitated per hundred spermatozoa. Leukocytes may resemble sperm precursors and should be differentiated from these immature germ cells. The relationship between leukocyte number and the presence of genital tract infection is unclear.

If the leukocyte count is very high, the ejaculate may appear yellowish–opaque. The condition is sometimes referred to as pyospermia. If pyospermia is present, the patient should be referred to a urologist.

Subfertile men often exhibit an increased number of leukocytes in their ejaculates and in their expressed prostatic fluid. Antibiotic treatment often decreases leukocyte number and significantly improves sperm motility.

Leukocytospermia may be considered a contributory subfertility factor, rather than a primary cause.

Erythrocytes

Erythrocytes (red blood cells) are typically not present in the healthy ejaculate. Their presence is usually due to a pathology in the reproductive tract, a condition referred to as hematospermia.

What is hematospermia?

Hematospermia or hemospermia is the presence of fresh or altered blood (erythrocytes) in the ejaculate.

How is it determined?

Pinkish or reddish discoloration of semen, or the presence of erythrocytes in microscopic examination of the semen specimen.

Significance

Hematospermia may be the result of inflammation, ductal obstruction or cysts, neoplasms, vascular abnormalities, systemic or iatrogenic factors. Of these, iatrogenic causes of hematospermia are most common.

Presence of erythrocyte does not appear to influence the absolute fertilizing potential of the spermatozoon. The overall incidence of hematospermia remains unknown.

Recommendation

Erythrocytes in the seminal fluid, while not affecting fertilizing potential, remain a cause for concern. Urological consultation is a must.

Epithelial cells

Significance

Some epithelial cells, possibly originating from the urethra or from the meatus and glans as contaminates during masturbation, may be present in the seminal fluid and are typically of no significance. The normal continuous process of desquamation of squamous epithelia usually culminates in cell nucleus loss as the epithelial cells die (are anucleated). Therefore, large anucleate bodies of residual cytoplasm may also be found in the ejaculate. Their significance remains unknown.

Recommendation

Many epithelial cells within the sample may indicate that collection was by coitus interruptus, or orally. These semen collection methods may sometimes compromise the sperm quantity and quality (See 'Sperm Motility,' page 47). Should that be the case, then alternative collection methods should be advised (See 'Semen collection,' page 15).

Microorganisms

What is it?

Microorganisms may be found in the ejaculate. Most of them are regarded as either commensals or contaminants. Large numbers of such organisms may indicate contamination or a genital tract infection.

How is it determined?

When large numbers of bacteria are observed in the stained semen preparation, a bacterial culture and antibiotic sensitivity determination is recommended. Seminal plasma has some anti-bacterial properties; therefore, a negative culture may not rule out infection. A semen culture following a fourfold dilution with sterile media is recommended to accurately determine status.

A more specific approach entails the 'Three culture method':
- First, obtain a culture from midstream urine.
- Second, obtain a culture from the ejaculate.
- Third, obtain the last culture from postmasturbation midstream urine.

If the ejaculate culture is positive and different from the first mid-stream urine culture, then genital tract infection is confirmed.

Significance

Microorganisms within the ejaculate, presenting an increase in leukocyte concentration yet no observable effect on sperm motility, may suggest contamination and are clinically not significant.

Recommendation

Large numbers of bacteria usually suggests an infection of the reproductive tract, almost exclusively the prostate. Advice should be sought from other specialized laboratories. If bacteria are present, then antibiotic treatment based on antibiotic sensitivity findings is recommended, especially if IUI is to be performed.

Cells of spermatogenic origin

What is it?

Sperm precursors include spermatids, spermatocytes and spermatogonia.

Significance

The presence of these cells is usually associated with below normal sperm count and abnormal sperm morphology, and may suggest an overall reduction in fertility potential. In acute distress situations such as fever, intoxications, exposure to radiation or cytotoxic drugs, an abnormal number of sperm precursors may be present in the ejaculate, prior to the patient becoming azoospermic (See 'Sperm concentration,' page 37).

Recommendation
Refer to urologist (a biopsy may reveal the extent of involvement) or to an assisted reproductive specialist.

Sperm agglutination

What is it?

'Sperm agglutination' is sperm clumping into aggregates.

How is it determined?

Assessed in wet microscopic smears.

Agglutination encompasses two types of clumping: non-specific and site-specific.

- Non-specific agglutination: Sperm cells adhere to various seminal debris, leucocytes or mucus threads, and various other non-sperm cellular elements.

- Site-specific agglutination: Sperm cells adhere to each other in a site-specific manner, such as head-to-head, head-to-tail, tail-to-tail, or any combination thereof.

Significance

Site-specific agglutination typically signifies an immunological cause, and should be noted (see 'Antisperm antibody tests,' page 65). Non-specific agglutination, depending on how extensive, might suggest an accessory sex gland infection (See 'Leukocytospermia,' page 31). However, merely a few clusters of immotile agglutinated sperm clinging to debris, mucus, etc. is of no clinical significance.

Recommendation

If immunological factors are involved, treat accordingly (See 'Antisperm antibody tests,' page 65).

Sperm concentration and sperm count

What are they?

Sperm concentration is the number of sperm per milliliter of seminal fluid. Sperm count is the total number of sperm per ejaculate.

How are they determined?

Several methods are available. The hemocytometer counting chamber and the Makler chamber are frequently used to estimate sperm concentration. These yield at best a reliable estimate of the sperm concentration. Computer-assisted image analysis methods typically used to estimate sperm motility can also provide estimates of sperm concentration. This method gives repeatable results, but is dependent on system parameter settings specifically programed for sperm identification. Variations between counts of up to 20%, especially when relative numbers are high, should be expected.

After counting spermatozoa number in a known volume, concentration per milliliter is then easily ascertained. The total spermatozoa number in the ejaculate (sperm count) is calculated as the product of sperm concentration and ejaculate volume.

Abnormalcy?

According to the *WHO Laboratory Manual* (1999), a man is oligozoospermic if the sperm concentration in his ejaculate is less than 20×10^6 per milliliter. For clinical purposes, however, semen concentration is differentiated into three useful categories to facilitate interpretation and diagnosis.

- A man is azoospermic if no sperm are present in the ejaculate.
- He is oligozoospermic if sperm concentration is less than 10.0×10^6 per milliliter.
- He is polyzoospermic if sperm concentration is more than 250×10^6 per milliliter.

Azoospermia diagnosis should be made only after an undiluted ejaculate is centrifuged, and the complete absence of spermatozoa in the centrifuge pellet is microscopically confirmed in not less than two ejaculates.

The differentiation between azoospermia and oligozoospermia is important clinically because azoospermia is very difficult, if not impossible, to treat, and the respective therapeutic recommendations vary greatly.

AZOOSPERMIA

Azoospermia is due to obstruction in the sperm delivery path, hormonal insufficiency, congenital factors, therapeutic factors, immunological factors, and idiopathic factors.

Obstruction of sperm delivery path

If due to the congenital absence of the vas deferens and seminal vesicles (as in cystic fibrosis) or ejaculatory duct obstruction, absence of fructose in the ejaculate (characteristic of seminal vesicle secretions) will prove diagnostically significant. Additionally, the ejaculate volume will be low with pH levels less than 7.4 (see 'volume,' page 26). By contrast, when obstruction at the epididymis is the apparent cause (usually the result of a sexually transmittable disease or rarely as in Young's Syndrome) fructose will be present, but α-glucosidase (produced by the epididymis) will be absent (See 'Chemical analysis of seminal plasma,' page 70).

Hormonal insufficiency

If due to hypogonadotropic hypogonadism, then the ejaculate volume will be low. The seminiferous tubular diameter will prove very small with no spermatogonial cells or Leydig cells. The patient will assuredly have other clinical symptoms to aid in the diagnosis.

Congenital factors

Chromosomal abnormalities such as Klinefelter's XXY syndrome, XYY syndrome and microdeletions in the AZF region of the Y chromosomes can result in azoospermia (see further). Klinefelter's Syndrome eventually leads to the disappearance of all germ and Sertoli cells. The tubules become fibrotic and hyalinized.

Cases of arrested spermatogenesis have been associated with reciprocal translocation between autosomes and the sex chromosomes. Physically normal patients may have chromosomal abnormalities which cause oligozoospermia or azoospermia.

Therapeutic factors

Chemotherapeutic agents such as cyclophosphamide, busulfan, chlorambucil, thiotepa, procarbazine, vincristine and methotrexate are known to cause germinal cell aplasia, leading to azoospermia. Similarly, sulfasalazine and colchicine treatment results in azoospermia. Exposure to ionizing radiation also damages the germinal cells.

Immunological factors

Viral infection (for example, mumps orchitis contracted as an adult) or a physical injury to the testes may disrupt the blood–testis barrier and expose the haploid spermatogenic cells to the circulatory system. These cells are identified as foreign antigens, against which antibodies are then produced. The antibodies then enter the testes, and destroy the spermatogenic cells, eventually resulting in azoospermia.

Idiopathic factors

Germinal cell aplasia due to Sertoli cells only: in this syndrome, follicular stimulating hormone levels will be high (more than twofold). These individuals are typically sterile. In approximately 40% of these patients, however, spermatogenic pockets can be identified by sectional biopsy. If spermatozoa are actually found, they can then be extracted and utilized for ICSI.

Spermatogenic maturation arrest, where spermatogenesis does not proceed beyond the primary spermatocyte, the secondary spermatocyte, or the spermatid. The spermatogenic arrest may be similar in all the tubules, but can vary from patient to patient. Causes are currently unknown.

OLIGOZOOSPERMIA

A patient should be considered oligozoospermic if his sperm concentration is less than 10.0×10^6 per milliliter (some laboratories now set this value at 5×10^6 per milliliter).

Oligozoospermia may be due to procedural causes, clinical factors, therapeutic factors or idiopathic factors.

Procedural causes

Initial semen fraction loss during collection. Also, too short a sexual abstinence period or partial ejaculation due to incomplete orgasmic reflex (see 'Volume,' page 26).

Clinical factors

Partial obstruction at the epididymis or at the ampulla (subsequent ejaculate within one half to one hour will yield a higher sperm count).

Partial retrograde flow of ejaculate due to incomplete bladder sphincter closure (See 'retrograde flow of semen,' page 27).

Hyperprolactinemia may interfere with cell division. In this instance, bromocriptin treatment usually increases sperm count.

Varicocele, cryptorchidism, diabetes mellitus and multiple sclerosis patients may become oligozoospermic.

Congenital factors

Microdeletions in the AZF region of the Y chromosomes can result in oligozoospermia (see further).

Therapeutic factors

Nitrofurantoin, oxymetholone, methyltestosterone, stanozolol and olsalazine treatment may result in oligozoospermia. The antihypertensive drug guanethidine affects sperm transport, which may also cause oligozoospermia.

Idiopathic factors

No causes can be identified for the oligozoospermia. However, those sperm which are present are usually fertile.

AZOOSPERMIA AND OLIGOZOOSPERMIA

Various causes of both azoospermia or oligozoospermia such as thermal stress, congenital factors, hormonal insufficiency, therapeutic factors, habitual factors, environmental pollutants:

Thermal stress

Decrease in sperm count usually starts within 30 days after the first acute high fever, and decreases to a zero count for up to 70 days or thereof. Such count reduction occurs independently of patient's apparent recovery.

Congenital factors

Azoospermia factor deletions on the long arm of the Y chromosome are associated with infertility (known as 'Y-deletion'). These deletions occur in about 12% of azoospermic men and about 7% of severely oligozoospermic men.

Hormonal insufficiency

Sperm may be present and the volume might or might not be low. The patient will no doubt have other clinical symptoms to aid in the diagnosis. An interesting, illustrative case report is presented below.

A case report: hypoandrogenism

A 28-year-old male evaluated for endocrine disorder and found to be hypoandrogenic (Testosterone 201 ng/deciliter and LH < 3 mIU/milliliter). The magnetic resonance imaging of the pituitary gland confirmed an empty sella syndrome with suprasellar cistern extending into the sella. Patient opted to cryopreserve his ejaculates prior to being treated with hormones.

His semen analysis on four different occasions appears below.

Ejaculate	Volume (ml)	Sperm concentration ($\times 10^6$/ml)	Sperm motility (%)
1	2.4	6.0	83
2	3.0	3.3	71
3	2.5	3.0	78
4	2.7	3.0	67

Even with such low testosterone and LH levels, reasonable quality and quantity of spermatozoa can be expected.

Therapeutic factors

Many drugs such as spironolactone, sulfasalazine, nitrofurantoin, niridadozole and colchicine are detrimental to spermatogenesis and sperm quality, significantly reducing male fertility potential.

Behavioral factors

Chronic alcoholism may interfere with the spermatogenic process and also damage the spermatozoa during epididymal transport.

Other ingested agents that may indirectly affect semen quality are nicotine, ethanol, marijuana, and morphine. These compounds affect the gonadal function or interfere with gonadotropin action. Anabolic hormones such as androgens can also affect spermatogenesis.

Environmental pollutants

Exposure to toxicants such as 1,2 dibromochloropropane-117 and ethylene dibromide also affect spermatogenesis. Compounds in the environment with estrogenic effects may also cause defects in spermatogenesis.

POLYZOOSPERMIA

Polyzoospermia is usually due to long sexual abstinence periods. Relatively high sperm concentrations of 700.0×10^6 spermatozoa per milliliter or more usually result in poor overall sperm quality. Fertility potential may also be compromised. Artificial insemination with processed sperm is advisable. (In this author's laboratory, the highest observed concentration of spermatozoa was 1.2×10^9 per milliliter of semen, and the ejaculate appeared milky white).

Significance

Sperm count alone, although a potentially determining factor, is not an accurate indicator of fertilizing potential. Only when azoospermic is it an absolute factor.

When donor sperm are utilized, spouses of azoospermic men conceive with greater 'facility' than spouses of oligozoospermic men. This clinical fact suggests that some spouses of oligozoospermic men often have some underlying subfertility cause of their own; otherwise, these women would have conceived on their own, with similar frequency to the spouses of azoospermic men.

Prevasectomy semen examination of 1890 men with children revealed that 8% had a sperm concentration of 5×10^6 spermatozoa per milliliter or less, about 16% had fewer than 10.0×10^6 per milliliter and about 25% had fewer than 20.0×10^6 per milliliter. Equating the prevasectomy semen to the ejaculate at conception is questionable. Such a conclusion is speculative, and the acceptance of present semen as a reasonable representation of the specimen at conception, while logical, is risky. However, a significant number of allegedly fertile men might actually have sperm counts that are clinically still considered oligozoospermic.

The determination of low fertility potential, based solely upon sperm count, is extremely uncertain. As long as a single spermatozoon is present in the ejaculate, the possibility for fertilization, however remote, nonetheless exists.

Almost every fertility specialist has encountered a patient with severe oligozoospermia who, to everyone's surprise, impregnated his spouse. The seemingly paradoxical fact remains: men with very low sperm counts often prove fertile. Patients treated for hypogonadotropic hypogonadism can display fertility, even when their sperm count may not exceed 1×10^6 per milliliter. Men on clinical trials with potential contraceptive agents remain fertile, even when their sperm counts appear substantially low. Thus, below average sperm production is compatible with fertility so long as overall sperm quality remains acceptable and no problems exist with their spouses' reproductive status.

Ambient temperature, even though relatively high, should not affect spermatogenesis (if temperature remains within a tolerable range). The human body's ability to thermoregulate core body temperature should provide an adequate compensatory effect. However, occupational exposure (such as a furnace or boiler room, the work-related thermal variation of fire fighters, professional cooks, truck and taxi drivers, etc.) may produce thermal stress sufficient for the debilitation of semen quality (see 'Sperm morphology,' page 51). Note that such factors as tight fitting underwear, saunas, prolonged immersion in hot water (whirlpool) baths and steam (Turkish) baths do not systematically seem to have the debilitating effects once thought.

Recommendation

Genetic screening for Y-deletions in men with oligozoospermia or azoospermia prior to TESE or MESA for ICSI is strongly recommended. These procedures regrettably enable the transmission of such genetic mutations to all sons born as a result of treatment. So, while most of the father's deletions are found to be de novo – and not inherited from the father – ICSI nonetheless make these mutations inheritable.

Overall sperm count and sperm concentration are both relevant factors; however, their clinical significance is based upon semen volume. For example, a patient might display extremely high sperm concentration with a very low semen volume, making overall sperm count below prescribed reference values. Therefore, the couple may remain infertile, necessitating artificial insemination techniques. Alternatively, sperm count may be adequate, but overall semen volume so high that sperm concentration falls below prescribed reference values. This may also affect fertility, also necessitating artificial insemination techniques.

Repeat semen analysis is recommended prior to definitive diagnosis. Once diagnosis is secured, then recommendations are as follows.

- If due to obstruction: refer to a urologist for evaluation and correction.
- If due to hormonal deficiency: refer to endocrinologist for hormonal treatment.
- If no treatment or surgical correction is feasible: process sperm for artificial insemination, or refer to an assisted reproductive specialist.

As a viable alternative, artificial insemination with donor sperm should be considered.

Sperm motility

What is it?

The observation of spontaneous sperm movement.

How is it determined?

The ratio of the number of motile sperm to total number of sperm (in a given volume), and is expressed as a percentage. Several techniques more objective than visual observation – including laser doppler velocimetry, spectrophotometry, photon correlation spectroscopy, and timed-exposure or multiexposure photomicrography – have been developed. Recently, much attention has been given to microcinematography, videomicrography, and computer-aided sperm analysis (CASA) for the determination of specific movement characteristics, such as tail amplitude and lateral head movement.

None of these newer and highly technical research procedures has found extensive clinical application until now. Moreover, such precise, complicated and costly methods have not proven effective in fertility diagnosis. Additionally, semen quality naturally varies significantly between two consecutive samples obtained within a short period, or between samples even when obtained over an extended period of time. Consequently, any measurement of motility, however accurate, may not provide any additional clinical advantage regarding semen quality. (As opposed to other sampling types, such as blood count or the determination of blood chemistries, where a small sample is extracted from a much larger, mostly homogeneous volume, and remains highly repeatable between samples.)

The visual estimation of sperm motility can vary by as much as 20%. Since precise motility determination is of relatively little value for fertility testing, such visual estimation, while subjective and not precise, nonetheless clinically suffices.

Abnormalcy?

According to the *WHO laboratory manual* (1999), a man is asthenozoospermic if the sperm in his ejaculate shows less than 50% forward progression within 60 minutes of ejaculation.

However, for clinical purposes, a man is asthenozoospermic if the sperm in his ejaculate shows less than 40% overall motility within 60 minutes of ejaculation and necrozoospermic if all spermatozoa are immotile.

Frequent ejaculation decreases spermatozoa number but does not seem to significantly impair percent motility. True necrozoospermia can be diagnosed only after performing the supravital (viability) stain (See 'Sperm membrane integrity test,' page 58). Immotile sperm does not imply dead sperm. A case report is presented below to elucidate the importance of identifying true necrozoospermia.

A case report: pregnancy with necrozoospermic ejaculate

A patient clinically evaluated for secondary infertility produced several ejaculates that were diagnosed necrozoospermic. His serum gonadotropins and testosterone were within normal limits and antisperm antibodies were negative:

Ejaculate	Sperm concentration ($\times 10^6$/ml)	Sperm motility	Sperm morphology
1	86.0	0	Normal
2	126.0	0	Normal
Spontaneous natural conception			
3	136.0	0	30

Further sperm studies revealed that 90 to 95% of his sperm were acrosome reacted. Freeze-fractured sperm analysis under electron microscopy revealed normal tail fibers and mitochondria. Sperm penetration test and hemizona binding test were also negative. Then, IVF was attempted, yet failed; ICSI, did produce embryos. However, during the couple's evaluation period, his spouse conceived following frequent sexual activity. Paternity testing confirmed this patient's status as the child's father.

All laboratory findings indicated that the sample, indeed, possessed zero fertility potential, the natural conception by his spouse incontrovertibly proved otherwise.

(Anecdotally, in the 1960s a bull exclusively produced sperm with no tails. Following multiple intrauterine insemination procedures, a cow successfully conceived. In such a non-human instance, motility was an absolute zero, yet in vivo conception still occurred.)

Overall, relating laboratory findings, no matter how accurately determined, to actual fertility potential of a given individual must be done with considerable caution.

Asthenozoospermia is due to procedural causes, congenital factors, clinical factors, immunological factors or idiopathic factors:

Procedural causes

These include psychological, physiological and methodological causes.

PSYCHOLOGICAL CONDITIONS AFFECT SPERM MOTILITY

Lack of adequate sexual stimulation during collection may also prove detrimental to sperm motility (see 'sexual stimulation,' page 15).

MANY PHYSIOLOGICAL FACTORS CAN AFFECT SPERM MOTILITY

Loss of the initial semen fraction during collection is an important factor. A majority of sperm and prostatic fluid are present in the initial fraction; the latter fraction, high in seminal vesicle fluid (which tends to have a deleterious effect on sperm motility) is lower in sperm number. For these reasons, the percentage of motile sperm and overall sperm survival are statistically better in the first fraction of a split ejaculate than in the entire semen sample. Long periods of abstinence before collection also prove detrimental to sperm motility.

METHODS OF SEMEN COLLECTION CAN ALSO AFFECT SPERM MOTILITY

Coitus withdrawal or oral collection may cause initial fraction loss. Dilution by acidic vaginal fluids or saliva can also influence sperm motility. Identification of either vaginal epithelial or buccal epithelial cells in the sample can confirm the method of collection. Similarly, overall semen volume can be unnaturally increased through the addition of those fluids.

Sperm motility might be affected during transport by exposure to cold, direct sunlight or excessive heat, etc.

COLLECTION CONTAINER WILL ALSO INFLUENCE SPERM MOTILITY

Containers utilized for sample collection and transport have included everything from tupperware to nursing bottles. They may have been cleaned with household soap and water, and, if not rinsed properly, will kill or injure sperm. Sterilization of containers by boiling and air drying can also prove detrimental to sperm since salt deposits from the water can alter semen pH and osmolality indirectly altering sperm motility.

Clinical factors

Male reproductive tract infection can create an increase of leukocytes that, in turn, produce by the generation of free oxygen radicals and the release of cytotoxic cytokine agents deleterious to sperm (see 'Leukocytospermia,' page 31). Pathological conditions accompanied by high fever may affect sperm motility.

Congenital factors

Deficiency of certain seminal glycoproteins may also affect sperm movement.

Kartagener's syndrome is a condition where the axonemal dynein complexes are either defective or absent, resulting in immotile sperm. Dyneins are large, multi-subunit ATPases that interact with microtubules in the tail to generate the force needed for sperm motility. These sperm are immotile, yet not necrozoospermic, since ICSI procedures using these sperm can yield successful pregnancies.

Immunological factors

Immunoglobulins may attach to the sperm membrane surface and either interfere with membrane function or influence the sperm motility by their physical presence on the spermatozoon.

Idiopathic factors

No known causes exist for asthenozoospermia. However, motile sperm from such specimens can be harvested and processed for artificial insemination.

Significance

Abnormal sperm (except for headless or 'pin-point' sperm) never show good motility; so good motility is therefore an inherent characteristic of good sperm. However, sperm with abnormal DNA content may look and behave like normal sperm, while exhibiting zero fertility potential. As a general rule, it could be stated that all fertile sperm are naturally motile (with some exceptions, as previously indicated) but not all motile sperm are naturally fertile.

Sperm motility is susceptible to temperature variation. Since even room temperature varies drastically even under laboratory conditions, (air conditioning, heating, or open windows, etc.) motility analyses should be performed under controlled thermal conditions, preferably corresponding to body temperature (37 °C).

Sperm motility is also time dependent and decreases over time, so that original percent motility can decrease by as much as 50% after 4 to 7 hours. Motility evaluation should therefore be conducted at a consistent and repeatable time period and temperature. For example, standardize the laboratory analysis, test for motility at 1 hour post ejaculation, and at a standardized room temperature.

'Progressive sperm motility' is a percentage of the number of motile sperm moving in a linear, forward progression. Progressive sperm motility should be at least 75% percent or more of the overall sperm motility. If asthenozoospermia is noted, then assess the progressive sperm motility. If the progressive sperm motility is 75% or more of the actual sperm motility, then one can suspect a problem with the transport or collection container (sperm motility of original sample was probably good, overall sperm motility therefore was affected by faulty sample transport).

Human IVF and zona free hamster egg penetration tests reveal that sperm motility alone is not a sufficient variable for fertility assessment. Also, improving the percentage of sperm motility alone does not cause a significant improvement in conception rates after IUI.

Motility is therefore only one of many variables influencing fertility; consequently, sperm motility must be extremely low to actually be the sole infertility cause.

Recommendation

Asthenozoospermia associated with a high concentration of leukocytes and seminal debris is suggestive of an accessory sex gland infection. In such an instance, a bacterial culture, followed by specific antibiotic treatment, is advisable.

If sperm concentration is in the acceptable range, morphologically normal spermatozoa is in the reference range (see further), and no leukocytes or other abnormalities are present, relatively low motility values remain acceptable.

Barely motile or completely immotile but not dead spermatozoa can still be utilized for artificial insemination after stimulating sperm activity by the application of additives. Typical additives recommended for the stimulation of sperm motility are 36 mmol caffeine in modified Ringer's buffer, 3×10^{-8} M kallikrein in saline, and 8 mmol L-arginine in saline. As a reminder, these compounds have not increased the fertilizing capacity of spermatozoa, only their motility. The initial differentiation between dead and immotile sperm is therefore of clinical importance.

Because dead or poorly motile spermatozoa affect fertilizing capacity of other spermatozoa, removal of these spermatozoa is useful prior to IUI or IVF. Techniques are available to separate motile from immotile spermatozoa, including 'swim-up,' colloidal suspension of silica particles or Nycodenz density gradient centrifugation, and glass (silica) wool or Sephadex column filtration methods. A number of andrologists recommend the use of motile sperm number rather than percent sperm motility as a fertility index. The usefulness of this parameter has yet to be clinically confirmed.

Sperm morphology

What is it?

Shape and appearance of spermatozoa.

How is it determined?

A semen smear is prepared on a glass slide, air dried, fixed, stained and examined at a magnification of at least 1000× under oil immersion bright field optics. Microscopic evaluations are subjective, and interpretations of abnormality vary according to the observer. New methodologies have been introduced to standardize morphological assessment, including the video overlay method and the semiautomatic/automatic image analysis system. The clinical usefulness of these techniques over standard methodology is currently uncertain. Preliminary data are not encouraging. Similarly, routine spermatozoon ultrastructure evaluation is neither practical nor clinically necessary. Scanning or transmission electron microscopy may be employed to identify specific spermatozoon structural abnormalities when considered important, but mostly are of academic interest.

Punctilious analysis of stained spermatozoa can identify many minor deviations from an otherwise 'perfect' sperm cell. If such detailed analysis reveals fewer than 15% 'normal' sperm, then the sample is of abnormal morphology. Such an assessment might prove valuable for IVF, but is questionable for routine sperm quality assessment.

Abnormalcy?

According to most publications, a man is teratozoospermic if the sperm in his ejaculate contains more than 70% abnormal forms. However, for clinical purposes (especially for the differential evaluation of sperm morphology), a man is teratozoospermic if his ejaculate displays more than 60% with abnormal morphology.

Teratozoospermia may be due to clinical factors, therapeutic factors, stress factors, or congenital factors

Clinical factors

FEVER

Any debilitating illness such as fever will produce an increase in abnormal sperm number. Increase in sperm with cytoplasmic droplets usually occurs within two weeks of acute manifestation, suggesting inadequate sperm maturation (which takes place in the epididymis, an organ sensitive to heat stress). Morphological abnormalities may continue to rise for up to 70 days or thereafter, even though the patient's clinical status may have improved. Morphological deviations include tapered sperm head, amorphous forms, and sperm precursors.

VARICOCELE

Varicocele is a condition that may increase abnormal sperm forms. Morphological deviations include amorphous forms and tapered spermatozoa, much more so than with infectious diseases. However, sperm function is more likely affected by varicocele than sperm morphology.

ALLERGIC REACTIONS

Morphological deviations include an increase in amorphous forms and sperm precursors, rather than tapered forms.

Therapeutic factors

Certain drugs that affect spermatogenesis (such as nitrofurans, including furadantin, an antibiotic used for treatment of urological infection), produce morphological alterations.

Stress factors

Persistent physical or psychological stress can also produce morphological deviations.

PHYSICAL

Testicular heat increase is considered a factor. Causes such as tight fitting underwear, hot baths, saunas, steam baths, etc., have been suggested; however, such factors and their effects on sperm morphology remain questionable.

PSYCHOLOGICAL

Emotional stress may play a similar role, but is equally questionable.

Congenital factors

Microdeletions in the AZF region of the Y chromosomes can result in teratozoospermia. Sperm may be also produced without an acrosome. To illustrate a true case of teratozoospermia, consider the following case report.

A case report: acrosomeless spermatozoa

Infertile for 7 years, the man produced ejaculates containing spermatozoa that were completely devoid of acrosome.

His semen analysis on two different occasions appears below.

Ejaculate	Volume (ml) (ml)	Sperm concentration $(\times 10^6/ml)$	Sperm motility (%)	Acrosomeless Sperm (%)
1	1.4	54.5	28	100
2	1.8	126.5	46	100

The vital staining yielded 72% unstained ('live') spermatozoa and the hypoosmotic swelling test resulted in 69% swollen spermatozoa. Transmission electron microscopy confirmed the absence of acrosome and postacrosomal sheath formation in all the sperm examined. The acrosin levels were decreased fivefold and the proacrosin levels were decreased almost eightfold as compared to normal values. Zona free hamster egg penetration test was negative.

This condition results in the inability of spermatozoa to penetrate the egg, making fertilization impossible. However, subsequent ICSI is reported to have been successful.

Significance

A particular diagnosis is justified when specific sperm abnormalities are demonstrated to occur frequently in the ejaculate, not just occasionally. Although specific morphological abnormalities are more common under particular clinical conditions, the efficacy of further subdivision is questionable.

A relatively high number of abnormal sperm forms are present in normal human semen. Although 60% abnormal sperm morphology indicates a testicular or epididymal impairment, fertility potential need not be compromised.

Recommendation

Morphological abnormalities must be extremely high in semen for fertility to be affected. Based on the sperm abnormality type, the recommendations are as follows.

- If varicocele is suspected as a causal agent: urological examination and management is recommended.
- If moderate teratozoospermia is confirmed: IUI following sperm selection to improve the sperm quality should be considered.
- If severe teratozoospermia is confirmed: IVF following sperm selection to improve the sperm quality or ICSI should be considered.
- If IVF and ICSI procedures are not available: artificial insemination with donor sperm should be considered.

SPECIALIZED SEMEN ANALYSIS

When the spouse is found to be normal (within range of existing diagnostic techniques), and if the standard semen analysis results are also within reference range, specialized tests are then recommended. Additionally, when the standard semen analysis results yield equivocal values (see Table 1) or are abnormal, specialized tests are also recommended.

These specialized tests are not routinely performed, and most of their reference values have yet to be firmly established. However, these tests can provide valuable diagnostic information concerning certain individuals.

Sperm function tests

The inherent ambiguity between sperm function and sperm property makes differentiation difficult, if not impossible. Clinical purpose and clarity demand that anything observed within, or evaluated about, an ejaculate constitutes a sperm property, such as motility. In contrast, any new observable sperm change or action induced by a particular stimulus, including an external factor or agent interaction, is classified as a sperm function. The following descriptions provide a logical array of 'sperm function tests'.

Spermatozoa may appear normal but may not be able to penetrate and migrate through the cervical mucus and consequently cannot reach the fertilization site. Such migratory capacity or incapacity can be tested by allowing the sperm to penetrate and move through cervical mucus in vitro.

The biochemical events that allow sperm to fertilize are collectively called capacitation (see 'Sperm–oocyte Interaction' page 18). Capacitation primarily involves changes in the sperm membrane system and is a process that occurs when sperm are in the female reproductive tract. The sperm membrane must be intact and functional for these events to occur. The spermatozoa structural and functional integrity may be evaluated by exposing them to a non-penetrating dye or hypoosmotic medium.

To determine whether sperm capacitation has occurred, an acrosome reaction can be induced artificially. Alternatively, sperm can be added to isolated human zona pellucida or to zona free hamster oocytes and extent of binding or penetration determined. If spermatozoa are capacitated, they will undergo the acrosome reaction and bind or penetrate oocytes.

Sperm mucus penetration test

What is it?

To reach the fertilization site, spermatozoa must penetrate and migrate through the cervix and the cervical mucus. Failure of in vitro penetration is often thought to imply failure in vivo.

How is it measured?

Human cervical mucus is not readily available for testing, and its properties can vary dramatically during the normal menstrual cycle. The presence of antibodies or white blood cells in cervical mucus may influence both spermatozoa migration and their survival.

Bovine cervical mucus or synthetic media are typically used. Although such animal and artificial systems differ from human cervical mucus, human spermatozoa appear to migrate into bovine and synthetic cervical mucus similarly as into human cervical mucus, confirming the viability of their use.

Abnormalcy?

Spermatozoa cannot adequately penetrate and migrate through cervical mucus.

Significance

Detailed sperm motion analysis may provide the same information as the mucus penetration test and, indeed, the test was shown to correlate with a number of sperm variables. However, men have been identified who exhibit poor sperm motility and low sperm concentration, but whose spermatozoa nonetheless show good mucus penetration and achieve natural fertilization. Actively motile spermatozoa with good forward progression typically score well in these tests, so this specialized test is predominantly useful only with already questionable samples.

Recommendation

If abnormal, IUI is recommended following sperm selection to improve the overall sperm quality.

Sperm membrane integrity test

What is it?

Membrane integrity is important to sperm success. Sperm motility, sperm capacitation, the acrosome reaction, and the binding of spermatozoon to egg surface can all be compromised should membrane integrity prove questionable or in any way inadequate. Thus, sperm membrane integrity and functionality is significant, and membrane function assessment may prove important in assessing sperm fertilizing capacity.

How is it determined?

Two tests are available to evaluate sperm membrane integrity: the supravital (viability, live–dead stain) and the hypoosmotic swelling (HOS) test.

The supravital stain determines whether the membrane is physically intact. When physically damaged or broken, the eosin Y dye is able to stain the sperm; if the membrane is intact, the dye is unable to do so. The stain thus evaluates the viablilty of a cell through the inclusion or exclusion of the eosin Y dye. Other viability stains are also available for this purpose. The percentage of viable spermatozoa as determined by the supravital stain should always be the same, or greater, than motile spermatozoa percentage.

Unlike the dye test, the HOS test determines sperm membrane functional integrity, through response to osmotic stress. Since the HOS test also reveals sperm percentage with a physically broken membrane, the supravital stain is therefore redundant. The sample is normal if the tested sperm shows more than 60% reactive ('swollen') spermatozoa.

Abnormalcy?

A sample is considered abnormal if more than 50% of the spermatozoa are stained or if less than 50% of sperm responds to the HOS test.

Significance

Within those normalcy parameters, the HOS test result is 75% to 85% predictive of the zona-free hamster penetration test outcome. More than 95% of prevasectomy ejaculates, which are presumably fertile, produce a normal HOS test response. By itself, the HOS test is a much better human IVF and in vivo conception predictor than standard semen analysis results. This test is also useful for the assessment of cryopreservation procedure membrane damage. However, one should be cautious, since only a single variable is measured: membrane function. Thus, the HOS test may give normal results for spermatozoa with zero fertility potential, since other, equally important, sperm variables such as acrosome integrity, might be overlooked.

Many embryologists now employ the HOS test to select sperm for ICSI.

Recommendation
If abnormal, IUI or IVF is recommended following sperm selection to improve sperm quality.

Sperm acrosome reaction test

What is it?

The acrosome reaction is an exocytotic event that occurs just prior to fertilization process. It involves the fusion of the outer acrosomal membrane with the surrounding plasma membrane, culminating in the acrosomal contents' release and dispersal.

How is it determined?

The sperm (capacitated) is mixed with inducers such as calcium ionophore A23187, progesterone, and intact or solubilized zona. The reaction is halted by fixative addition. The acrosomal status is then evaluated by an accepted technique, such as double staining or the PSA fluorescent stain technique. If 9% to 12% of sperm undergo acrosome reaction following induction, then the sample is considered normal. Presently, no clinical consensus exists as to indicators of overall test validity.

Abnormalcy?

Most sperm within an ejaculate have undergone acrosome reaction prematurely (see 'A case report: pregnancy with necrozoospermic ejaculate' page 48) or cannot be induced to undergo the acrosome reaction (see 'a case report acrosomeless spermatoza,' page 53).

Significance

The capacity for spermatozoa to undergo the acrosome reaction is measured directly by acrosome functional activity. Sperm populations that do, or do not, fertilize human oocytes in vitro display no significant differences in their ability to undergo spontaneous acrosome reaction. Spermatozoa with poor fertilizing potential display significantly less induced acrosome reaction than fertile sperm. Thus, the induced acrosome reaction may be a useful acrosomal function indicator; however, more studies are required before clinical use is recommended and functional parameters determined.

Recommendation

If abnormal, ICSI is recommended, when ICSI is not available artificial insemination with donor sperm should be considered.

Hemizona or zona binding test

What is it?

Spermatozoon ability to bind to the outer surface of zona pellucida, a prerequisite prior to binding and penetrating the egg vitelline membrane.

How is it determined?

The spermatozoon binding activity can be tested by using either non-living, intact human oocytes, or isolated zonae obtained from autopsy-derived ovaries, from surgically excised ovarian tissue, or from immature or surplus unfertilized oocytes during IVF.

The salt-stored oocytes are washed and either the whole or microbisected hemizonae incubated with capacitated sperm droplets. Sperm tightly bound to the zona pellucida outer surface are counted.

Abnormalcy?

Sperm that do not bind or exhibit a low number of sperm (poor) binding to the zona pellucida.

Significance

More than 90% of the tightly zona bound sperm undergo the acrosome reaction, so that this test can be used to evaluate spermatozoa undergoing this reaction.

Test results have 95% sensitivity and 83% specificity and a positive and negative predictive value for IVF outcome of 95% and 83% respectively.

Few laboratories presently perform the hemizona or zona binding test. Although results are interesting and warrant further investigation, human zonae acquisition is a major problem, making routine testing highly unlikely. The test is also labor intensive, lacks good quality control, and requires experienced and well-trained personnel.

If abnormal binding occurs, then the infertility cause may be identified. This assay is a valuable tool in identifying patients who may benefit with ICSI over IVF.

Recommendation

If abnormal, ICSI is recommended. If ICSI is not available, then artificial insemination with donor sperm should be considered.

Sperm penetration test

What is it?

Normal spermatozoa can bind and penetrate the egg vitelline membrane, a prerequisite to fusion with the egg contents

How is it determined?

Zona free (denuded) hamster eggs will allow capacitated sperm from other species to bind and penetrate the egg. This phenomenon is utilized to evaluate fertility potential of human spermatozoa.

Zona free hamster oocytes are added to capacitated sperm droplets and incubated for 2 to 3 hours. Following incubation, the oocytes are examined microscopically for sperm penetration. Penetration is judged to have occurred if either a swollen sperm head or a male pronucleus with a corresponding sperm tail is found within the hamster's ooplasm. The percentage penetration is taken as oocyte number penetrated, divided by total oocyte number examined, times 100.

Abnormalcy?

If sperm accomplish no penetration, or insignificant number of oocytes are penetrated.

Using TEST-yolk medium with cold storage technique for this evaluation, abnormal cut-off is taken as less than 10 percent penetration. Some laboratories only consider 0% penetration as abnormal. Few andrologists use the 'optimized' sperm penetration test. Here the fertile male exhibits extensive polyspermy with all ova penetrated. Less than five sperm penetrated per egg is considered poor for IVF; however, not for in vivo fertilizing capacity.

Significance

The test is useful, but the data need to be interpreted with care and should be considered only in conjunction with the other sperm test results. When no or poor penetration occurs, the test should always be repeated (possibly under different conditions) before reaching a definite conclusion. SPA implementation as a routine laboratory test is hindered by potential pitfalls, such as technical difficulties, relatively poor repeatability, and variable techniques employed by numerous laboratories. In addition, leukocyte presence can adversely affect the test outcome. The test is labor intensive, lacks good quality control, and requires experienced and well-trained personnel.

Recommendation
If deemed abnormal after at least two different tests, IVF is recommended following sperm selection to improve the sperm quality, with ICSI as a backup. If IVF is not available, then artificial insemination with donor sperm should be suggested.

What is it?

The quality of the haploid number of chromosomes in the sperm nucleus.

How is it determined?

Chromatin stability can be assessed directly by staining with aniline blue, or by assessing the swollen nuclei percentage following treatment with chemicals or heat. Chromatin condensation degree can be estimated by acridine orange staining.

Abnormalcy?

Increased chromatin instability and poor chromatin condensation is associated with reduced sperm fertility potential.

Significance

During spermatogenesis's later stages, the lysine-rich nucleoprotein histones are replaced by much more basic protamines such as arginine and cysteine. The protamines pack the DNA tightly into highly condensed chromatin, so that the sperm nucleus has extraordinary stability. Lack of normal chromatin condensation indicates developmental abnormalities, and may be associated with infertility.

Recommendation

Normal chromatin condensation and the sperm nucleus stability indicate developmental normalcy, and any deviation may be associated with infertility. Limited studies in humans and bulls have shown an association between sperm chromatin stability and fertility. Further studies in humans need to validate these determinations; appropriate recommendations require future validation.

What is it?

Spermatozoa are antigenic. When the immune reacting cells in the circulatory system are exposed (come into contact) with sperm, the body responds by producing antibodies against the sperm. Antisperm antibodies primarily cause sperm agglutination, immobilization or surface bound, and may be a cause of infertility in 12% to 20% of couples who have no other demonstrable explanations.

How is it measured?

Many different methods are available for evaluation of antisperm antibodies in blood, seminal plasma, spermatozoa, and cervical mucus. Methods that test for serum antisperm antibodies are referred to as indirect tests, while tests for antibodies on patients' spermatozoa are called direct tests.

Agglutination methods

The available tests are: gelatin agglutination test (Kibrick method), Tube-slide agglutination test (F–D method), tray agglutination test (Friberg method), capillary tube agglutination test (Shullman–Hekman method), or slide agglutination test.

These tests all yields a titer at which the agglutinating antibody is present

Immobilization methods

Sperm immobilization test – Isojima method
This test yields a positive or negative result.

Surface-bound antibody methods

Radio-labeled immunoglobulins, immunoglobulins, mixed antiglobulin test, or immunobeads (polyacrylamide spheres with covalently bound rabbit antihuman immunoglobulins)

These tests yield a percentage of sperm with surface-bound antibody.

Abnormalcy?

Antisperm antibody presence is due to infection, injury, vasectomy or idiopathic factors:

Infection

Urogenital system bacterial infections may also cause sperm agglutination, probably due to some common antigenic site shared by the sperm and the most common bacteria (staphylococcus).

Antibody directed spermatogenesis destruction due to mumps can result in azoospermia (see 'Sperm concentration and sperm count,' page 37).

Injury

Sperm are separated from the body's immune system by the blood–testis barrier and the blood–epididymal barrier. A physical injury that can lead to inflammation of the testis, causing the blood–testis barrier to break down, can lead to immune reacting cells to contact spermatozoa and other cells of spermatogenic origin. An antibody response is thus produced.

Vasectomy

About 60% of vasectomized men display antisperm antibodies in their blood. The surgically imposed obstruction at the vas deferens leads to increased back pressure at the rete testis region. Such pressure at a relatively weak region can lead to gradual sperm leakage. As the sperm enter the bloodstream, antisperm antibodies are induced.

Idiopathic factors

No known causes exist to explain the presence of antisperm antibodies.

Significance

The majority of men who actually possess antisperm antibodies in seminal plasma may still test negative with the indirect test. Consequently, whenever indirect tests are ordered, direct testing is also advisable.

Agglutination has also been observed with di- and trivalent salts, and with antihistamines.

Thus, sperm agglutination is not sole or absolute evidence for the presence of antisperm antibodies.

Sperm antibodies may interfere with spermatogenesis and sperm maturation in the male, and hinder sperm transport, cervical mucus penetration, capacitation, and fertilization in the female. Antisperm antibodies may also hinder spermatozoon fertilizing capacity.

A wide variation exists between different antisperm antibody tests. Test combinations may be able to reduce this inter test variation, and allow for more reliable interpretation and management of infertile patients who demonstrate antisperm antibodies.

Recommendations

Much confusion exists regarding antibody test interpretation because a direct correlation between sperm antibodies and infertility does not exist. Antibody presence probably indicates a genital tract disturbance, which may be the primary cause of infertility or subfertility, rather than the antibodies themselves. At present, prevalent sperm antibodies should be taken as an indication that immunologic problems may exist. In some cases, these antibodies can account for fertility problems, but in other cases, they are only contributory. Treatment modalities should take this into consideration.

▶ If the antibody titer or percent surface-bound antibody is low: immunological infertility is not the cause, and fertility prognosis is good.

▶ If the antibody titer or percent surface-bound antibody is moderate: immunological infertility is a suspect, and sperm should be processed for artificial insemination. A low dose prednisone treatment may decrease the immune response and aid in the removal of antisperm antibodies during sperm processing.

▶ If the antibody titer or percent surface-bound antibody is high: immunological infertility is one of the causes. IVF or ICSI is recommended. If these are unavailable, then artificial insemination with donor sperm should be suggested.

Acrosin, creatine phosphokinase and reactive oxygen species

What is it?

Egg outer layers penetration during fertilization is by enzymes such as acrosin, located in the sperm head. Acrosin has an essential role in acrosome reaction and in penetration through outer egg investments.

Many sperm metabolic activities and functions are controlled by enzymes and metabolites. Creatine phosphokinase is a key enzyme in energy synthesis and transport. Adenosine triphosphate, a metabolite, is essential for tail motion and several other sperm processes. Both these can be used as biochemical markers for midpiece activity.

Many biochemicals such as the reactive oxygen species, from the sperm and leukocytes, may interfere with sperm function. Oxidative stress has been reported to be an important cause of male infertility.

How is it determined?

Biochemical analysis involves either extraction or activation, followed by optical density change determination.

Abnormalcy?

Acrosin activity is low (<14 μIU/10^6 spermatozoa), activity of creatine phosphokinase is high (>0.250 CK Units/10^8 spermatozoa), or the reactive oxygen species amount is high ($>100 \times 10^4$ photons/minute/20×10^6 spermatozoa).

Significance

Sperm acrosome has an essential function in the fertilization process, it contains enzymes that are involved in the acrosome reaction, sperm binding to the zona pellucida, and spermatozoon penetration through the zona pellucida.

Acrosome chemical component intactness is essential for diagnostic purposes. For instance, ejaculates have been identified with reasonable sperm motility, but spermatozoa lacking acrosome have a very low acrosin content, and do not penetrate zona free hamster oocytes and are sterile (see 'A case report: acrosomeless spermatozoa,' page 53). Finally, acrosin assay can be used to identify infertile male subpopulations that would not be detected by physical sperm parameters.

Creatine phosphokinase activity is increased in infertile spermatozoa, probably due to increase in cytoplasmic proteins, suggesting a developmental defect. Incomplete cellular maturity could therefore be a testicular sperm maturation chemical marker. Although creatine phosphokinase activity has been reported to be a useful marker for sperm fertilizing capacity, further studies are necessary.

No energy sources such as adenosine triphosphate are presently utilized for diagnostic purposes, and will not be considered.

Unstable free oxygen radicals, such as those present in hydrogen peroxide, the hydroxyl radical and the superoxide anion are known as reactive oxygen species. These species are indigenous to spermatozoa, and take part in signal transduction. However, lipid peroxidation of the polyunsaturated fatty acids in the sperm membrane can be caused by elevated species levels, causing sperm dysfunction. Leukocytes within the semen produce reactive oxygen species that contribute to spermatozoon oxidative stress.

Recommendation

When abnormal levels are diagnosed, prognosis is poor. However, no clinical consensus as to the validity and relative severity of these assays exists at present. If any one of these three assays reveals an abnormal value, ICSI is recommended. If ICSI is unavailable, then artificial insemination with donor sperm should be suggested.

Infertile men empirically treated with antioxidants have demonstrated improved semen characteristics, improved fertilization in vitro, and, in one study, a higher fertility potential. Consequently, antioxidants also appear to play a role in sperm function and male infertility. The apparent link between oxidative stress and infertility suggests that antioxidant supplements might improve fertility potential.

Zinc, fructose, and α-glucosidase

The seminal vesicles, prostate and epididymis produce components quite specific for each accessory gland. These components are probably non-essential for sperm function, so their usefulness as fertility indicators is limited. However, these components assist in assessing accessory sex gland status. Accessory sex gland secretions can vary from ejaculate to ejaculate. Therefore, determination of the relative quantities present in semen is sufficient, except when the concentration of one component is radically low, implying a causal factor leading to compromised secretory function.

Although many components are produced by each accessory sex gland, some are non-specific, i.e. produced by other accessory sex glands. Therefore, the analysis of one component unique to each of the three major accessory sex glands or organ is sufficient for an overall estimation of accessory sex gland function.

What is it?

The chemical and enzymatic analysis of seminal plasma.

How is it determined?

Certain components are produced by a particular gland, such as fructose by the seminal vesicles, and zinc by the prostate gland, and α-glucosidase by the epididymis (see 'Semen component point-of-origin,' page 79).

All chemical and enzymic analyses involve either extraction and determination by optical density.

Abnormalcy?

Absence of seminal vesicle secretion is apparent if the ejaculate fails to coagulate, contains no fructose, has a pH below 7.2, and has reduced volume. (The ejaculate may or may not contain spermatozoa.)

If the ejaculate actually contains spermatozoa, the seminal vesicle ducts are probably occluded. To illustrate such an instance, consider the following case report.

A case report: obstruction at the colliculus seminalis

A 30-year-old male with unremarkable medical history, except for occasional hematospermia (suggestive of seminal vesiculitis) was evaluated for infertility. The patient also had a moderate bilateral varicocele, and produced several ejaculates for analysis. His serum gonadotropins and testosterone were within normal levels, and his antisperm antibodies were negative.

His semen analysis appears below.

Ejaculate	Volume (ml)	Sperm concentration ($\times 10^6$/ml)	pH	Zinc (mM)	Fructose (mM)
1	0.6	29.5	7.0		
2	0.9	35.0	7.3		
3	0.5	24.8	7.4	9.33	0
4	0.6	15.8			
5	0.8	0	7.0	11.63	
6	0.5	0		13.16	0.44

Seminal vesicles on vasogram were dilated, revealing no clear presence of the ejaculatory duct, indicating a partial obstruction.

Absence of fructose along with vasogram findings confirmed obstruction of the seminal vesical opening. The patient progressively became azoospermic as the apparent obstruction enlarged during the course of approximately 1 year.

Sperm may still be present in the semen, even with an obstruction at the colliculus seminalis. Therefore, hypospermic patients with sperm in their ejaculates, especially with low or no fructose levels and low pH (below 7.4), should have their seminal vesicles periodically examined. If left unchecked, azoospermia may result, with progressive and eventual complete obstruction at the ejaculatory duct. Semen cryopreservation is advisable.

If the ejaculate is azoospermic, then the vas deferens and seminal vesicles are likely to be congenitally absent, or the ejaculatory duct is totally occluded. To illustrate such an instance, consider the following case report.

A case report: congenital absence of seminal vesicle and vas deferens

An apparently healthy male with primary infertility produced several ejaculates for analysis. His serum gonadotropins and testosterone were within normal limits and antisperm antibodies were negative.

His semen analysis on two different occasions appears below.

Ejaculate parameters of a patient with congenital absence of seminal vesicle

Ejaculate	Volume (ml)	Sperm concentration ($\times 10^6$/ml)	pH	Zinc (mM)	Fructose (mM)
1	0.3	0	6.5	6.89	0.83
2	0.3	0	6.5		

Semen pH of 6.5 suggests a prostatic fluid with no contribution from the seminal vesicle gland. The chemical markers such as zinc for the prostatic gland and fructose for the seminal vesicular gland suggested an occlusion or aplasia of the vas deferens and seminal vesicle.

The vasogram confirmed the occlusion or aplasia of the ampulla. Testicular biopsy showed normal spermatogenesis, in turn confirming the diagnosis based on chemical analysis of the seminal plasma.

Reduced amounts or the complete absence of zinc is indicative either of possible initial fraction loss of the ejaculate during collection, or prostatic abnormality (see 'Volume,' page 26).

Seminal plasma chemical composition can be affected by other clinical and therapeutic factors:

Clinical factors

Diabetes can increase the seminal fructose concentration twofold.

Hypoandrogenism seminal volume and its chemical components will be reduced.

Therapeutic factors

Certain drugs may also influence seminal fluid composition. For example, thioridazine, phenoxybenzamine, and guanethidine inhibit accessory sex gland secretory activity.

Significance

Seminal component analysis allows an estimation of individual accessory sex gland or organ contribution to the entire ejaculate. The relative contribution of these chemicals and their evaluation can prove diagnostically useful.

These accessory sex gland components, however, have no association with spermatozoa fertilizing capacity.

Recommendation

If seminal plasma chemical composition abnormalities are observed, refer to a urologist for evaluation and eventual correction or to an assisted reproductive specialist for IVF or ICSI procedure.

pH

What is it?

Hydrogen ion concentration (reciprocal logarithmic expression of hydrogen ion concentration), and is a measure of alkalinity (pH > 7.0) and acidity (pH < 7.0).

How is it determined?

pH meter or pH paper indicator strips. Semen pH depends mainly on the relation between seminal vesicle alkaline secretion (pH 8.2 to 8.6) and prostate acid secretion (pH 6.8 to 7.2), and is slightly alkaline (pH 7.6 to 8.6). pH is also time dependent.

Abnormalcy?

According to *WHO Laboratory Manual* (1999), a reference value for semen pH is 7.2 or more; however, for clinical purposes to facilitate interpretation and diagnosis, semen pH of less than 7.6 or more than 8.6 is considered abnormal.

Abnormalities in pH may be due to clinical or procedural factors:

Clinical factors

Chronic prostatitis often displays a low pH (below 7.2), while acute prostatitis reveals a high pH (above 8.6).

Low semen volume, accompanied by low pH (below 7.2), is often due to a deficiency in seminal vesicle fluid (see 'A case report: obstruction at the colliculus seminalis,' page 71; and 'A case report: congenital absence of seminal vesicle and vas deferens,' page 72).

Low semen volume, accompanied by high pH (above 9.0), is often due to prostate gland pathology. To illustrate such an instance, consider the following case report.

A case report: diagnosis of prostatic cancer

An apparently healthy 49-year-old patient with secondary infertility, provided ejaculates for sperm processing and artificial insemination.

His semen analysis appears below.

Ejaculate parameters of a patient with prostatic cancer

Ejaculate	Volume (ml)	Sperm concentration ($\times 10^6$/ml)	Sperm motility (%)	pH
1	0.4	85.7	37	>9.0
2	0.3	70.0	9	
3	0.3	82.0	1	>9.0

Urological examination revealed a non-symptomatic advanced stage of prostatic cancer confirmed by biopsy (notice pH level of 9.0).

Procedural factors

Longer semen incubation will result in high pH (above 8.6) due to amines and amides breakdown. Initial fraction loss during collection may have higher pH (above 8.6). The sperm quantity and quality will usually be low, also.

Significance

The pH of semen is significant in human ejaculate analysis. Note that semen pH has little direct significance to sperm fertility potential, unless levels are excessively abnormal.

Recommendation

If pH abnormalities and seminal plasma chemical composition abnormalities are observed, refer to a urologist for evaluation and correction, or to an assisted reproductive specialist for IVF or ICSI procedure.

The logical sequence of routine and specialized semen analysis

To facilitate the understanding of concepts pertaining to the rationale for semen analysis and sperm function and their interpretation, the following narrative outline is provided:

Fertilization involves direct sperm-egg union. Essentially, sperm must be able to reach the fertilization site (possess adequate sperm motility and sperm morphology). Sperm must also be in sufficient numbers within the semen (sperm concentration) to overcome the statistical improbabilities of finally reaching the egg. The first obstacle in the female reproductive system is the cervical mucus. Sperm must penetrate and migrate through the cervical mucus (evaluated by a sperm mucus penetration assay).

Sperm, during passage through the female reproductive system, must undergo membrane alteration known as sperm capacitation. Once the sperm reach the egg, the spermatozoa must undergo further membrane alteration leading to acrosome reaction, which is dependent on the functional integrity of the membrane itself (evaluated by a hypoosmotic swelling assay). Sperm must then bind and penetrate the zona pellucida (evaluated by a hemizona assay) prior to fusing with the egg's vitelline membrane (evaluated by a sperm penetration assay).

According to the prescribed sperm function sequence, male fertility potential can best be evaluated in a similarly logical and sequential manner. In summary, the following panel of tests are suggested:

Sperm quality panel

Are the spermatozoon able to reach the fertilization site? Routine semen analysis and a satisfactory post-coital test or sperm mucus penetration assay are tests which enable that determination.

Sperm function panel

Are the spermatozoon able to fertilize an egg? Hypoosmotic swelling assay, hemizona assay and sperm penetration assay allow that determination.

Antisperm antibody test panel

Are immunological factors suspected? Antisperm antibodies have been implicated in 10–20% of unexplained infertility cases. Such a test panel should assess all three effects of antisperm antibodies (sperm agglutination, sperm immobilization and sperm surface binding).

Chemical analysis of seminal plasma panel

Based on preliminary semen analysis, do chemical components need to be assessed? Such a panel assesses fluid contribution from the epididymis, seminal vesicle, and prostate. The pH level is also determined.

Additional tests

Which other tests are required? Based on semen analysis, overall medical history and clinical findings from the spouse, other special testing such as spermatozoon ultrastructural evaluation, nuclear integrity assessment, biochemical analysis of spermatozoa, karyotyping, microdeletion in the Y chromosome determination or any other sophisticated sperm assays should be conducted, as indicated.

Semen component point-of-origin

Semen is composed of various elements, contributed by various organs and glands of the male reproductive tract. The following table graphically illustrates the clinically useful origins of these various components.

Interrelationship between semen characteristics and reproductive organelles

	Testis	Epididymis	Seminal vesicle	Prostate
Semen				
Coagulation			✗	✗
Liquefaction			✗	✗
Volume	✗	✗	✗	✗
Immunoglobulins		✗?	✗	✗
Leukocytes		✗?	✗	✗
Erythrocytes			✗	✗
Spermatozoa				
Count	✗			
Motility	✗	✗	✗	✗
Morphology	✗	✗		
Seminal plasma				
pH			✗	✗
α-glucosidase		✗		
Fructose			✗	
Zinc				✗

Conclusion

A major problem in semen analysis interpretation has been equating 'abnormal' with 'infertile' or 'subfertile' results. A semen variable abnormality simply means that it deviates from the average (normal) range. For example, consider the *WHO Laboratory Manual* (1999) standard reference values. Such a deviation may, or may not, cause infertility, depending on magnitude of severity and the fertility status of the spouse. A fertility problem does not exist simply because a semen variable is in an abnormal range, exemplified when overall semen quality can vary markedly between two consecutive ejaculates from the same individual. Also, some abnormalities have a greater effect on fertility than others. To avoid such confusion, we have now added a 'grey' (suspect) range of values to each variable and suggest terms such as 'usual,' 'equivocal,' and 'unusual' (see Table 1–3). Even so, abnormal and even unusual does not mean infertile, so that an abnormal (unusual) ejaculate differs from a normal (usual) ejaculate only in that it has less likelihood of being infertile (unless the other characteristics are extremely poor). Unfortunately, the relative fertility potential is often of little interest to a clinician who wants to know whether the patient has an overall fertility problem or not.

Since the term 'abnormal' is rather meaningless from a fertility standpoint, cutoff should be determined for each semen indicator (reference value) below a 95% infertility certainty. More information is required to establish firmly such 'infertility' values for these indicators. When one or more indicator falls into this infertility category, the ejaculate is almost certainly infertile. If no indicator falls into this category, a definitive diagnosis cannot be reached. Whenever indicators fall into the questionable, borderline category, such a phrase as 'less likely to be fertile' is applicable.

In every section, discussions and recommendations have been made regarding particular sperm parameters and their likely diagnosis. A vital element of such analyses involves consideration of the female. For example, sperm capacitation and acrosome reaction is as much dependent upon the female reproductive tract as inherent sperm quality. Consequently, sperm diagnosis might be qualified as 'normal,' yet the couple still may not conceive, due to ignorance of female reproductive tract problems or incompatibilities. Such a scenario can be confirmed when either the couple successfully conceives through IVF, or if the male, after changing partners, is able to impregnate his new spouse.

Sperm fertility assay interpretation is further complicated when dealing with assisted reproductive techniques. The semen analysis interpretation applicable to one particular technique may not be appropriate for another. For example, different sperm parameters are needed for ICSI, as compared to IVF or in vivo fertility are considered. Consequently, interpretation of semen analysis results is also subject to applied fertilization technique.

The dichotomy between 'diagnosis' and 'recommendation' is a critical one. Whereas the correct diagnosis might be obtained, the recommendation for that particular couple is dependent upon many variables. These include female fertility status, age of the female, emotional, ethical and financial factors. Given such sociological complexity in the treatment of infertility, a comprehensive guide to semen analysis interpretation can hopefully assist in the prognosis and management of the infertile male.

Table 1. Standard semen variable reference values for clinical interpretation and diagnosis

		Reference values		
	Results	Normal (usual)	Equivocal (grey)	Abnormal (unusual)
Macroscopic analysis				
Complete liquefaction (min)		60	60–120	120
Color: Pearl white, yellow, reddish		PW to Y	N/A	R/Other
Viscosity: normal, slight, marked		N	S	M
Volume (ml)		1.0–6.0	0.5–0.9	<0.5 or >6
Microscopic analysis				
Agglutination		0	1–2	>2
Leukocytes/400 HPF		<5	6–9	>10
Sperm concentration (10^6/ml)		≥20	10–19	<10
Sperm count (10^6/ejaculate)		≥50	20–49	<20
Physiological analysis				
Overall sperm motility (%)		≥40	35–39	<35
Progressive sperm motility (%)[a]				
Morphological analysis				
Normal sperm morphology (%)		≥40	35–39	<35
Abnormal sperm head (%)		<20	20–30	>30
Amorphous form (%)		<15	15–20	>20
Mid piece abnormal (%)[a]				
Tail abnormal (%)[a]				
Tapered form (%)[a]				
Others (%)[a]				

Note: [a] At present, no accepted reference values are available.

Table 2. Specialized semen test reference values for clinical interpretation and diagnosis

	Results	Reference values		
		Normal (usual)	Equivocal (grey)	Abnormal (unusual)
Mucus penetration				
Penetrak (mm/90 min)		≥ 30	20–29	<20
Membrane integrity				
Dye exclusion test:				
Sperm unstained by eosin-Y (%)		≥ 60	50–59	<50
Hypoosmotic swelling (HOS) test:				
Sperm responding to HOS test (%)		≥ 60	50–59	<50
Acrosome reaction assay				
Acrosome reacted sperm (%)[a]		≥ 9	5–9	<5
Zona free hamster assay				
Standard processing (%)		≥ 10	1–9	<1
TEST-yolk processing (%)		≥ 20	1–19	<1
Zona binding assay				
Hemizona binding		≥ 20	10–19	<10
Nucleus integrity tests				
Normal chromatin condensation[a]				
Stability of sperm DNA[a]				
Immunological analysis				
Sperm agglutination antibody test		$<1{:}20$	1:40	$>1{:}40$
Sperm immobilization antibody test		<2	2.0–2.5	>2.5
Indirect immunobead test (%)		<20	21–50	>50
Direct immunobead test (%)		<20	21–50	>50

Note: [a] At present, only preliminary or no accepted reference values are available.

Table 3. Spermatozoa biochemical analysis and seminal plasma chemical analysis reference values for clinical interpretation and diagnosis

	Results	Reference values		
		Normal (usual)	Equivocal (grey)	Abnormal (unusual)
Biochemical analysis				
Acrosin μIU/10^6sperm		>20	14–20	<14
Creatine phosphokinase CK units/10^8 sperm[a]		>0.250		
Reactive oxygen species[a] photons/minute/20×10^6 sperm		>100×10^4		
Chemical analysis				
pH		7.6–8.2	8.2–8.6	<7.6 >8.6
Total zinc (mM)		1.5–3.8	0.8–1.5	<0.8 >3.8
Fructose (mM)		>5.5	2.8–5.5	<2.8
α-glucosidase mIU/ejaculate		>20	10–20	<10

Note: [a] At present, only preliminary or no accepted reference values are available.

Glossary

Diagnostic terminology

Semen volume

Aspermia: no semen or fluid is emitted or obtained

Hypospermia: less than 0.5 milliliter semen

Hyperspermia: more than 6.0 milliliter semen

Sperm concentration

Azoospermia: no spermatozoa in the fluid

Oligozoospermia: less than 10×10^6 spermatozoa/milliliter

Polyzoospermia: more than 250×10^6 spermatozoa/milliliter

Sperm quality

Normozoospermia: between 20 and 250×10^6 spermatozoa/milliliter with more than 40% sperm motility and normal sperm morphology respectively

Sperm motility

Asthenozoospermia: less than 40% motility

Necrozoospermia: absence of sperm motility

Sperm morphology

Teratozoospermia: more than 60% of abnormal spermatozoa

Oligoasthenozoospermia, Oligoasthenoteratozoospermia or other combinations signifies various disturbance among the variables listed above.

Artificial insemination (AI)

The term artificial insemination was used by fertility specialists to distinguish between intercourse and the laboratory insemination process. The acronym *AI* was assigned to this procedure. Since AI is feasible with spouse or even donor sperm, the acronyms later became *AIH (artificial insemination with husband sperm)* or *AID (artificial insemination with donor sperm)*. After AIDS became recognized as a disease, the term AID obviously lost popularity. Instead, fertility specialists now use the term *TID (therapeutic insemination with donor sperm)*, or *TDI (therapeutic donor insemination)*.

When the semen, contained in a cap, is placed over the cervix, the procedure is referred to as *pericervical insemination (CAP insemination)* or when it is placed directly within the cervix, the procedure is referred to as *intracervical insemination (ICI)*.

When sperm is isolated from semen and placed within the uterus directly through the cervix, the procedure is referred to as *intrauterine insemination (IUI)*. If sperm is placed inside the fallopian tube, the procedure is referred to as *fallopian sperm perfusion (FSP)*.

Assisted reproductive technology (ART)

These include procedures to assist infertile couple achieve a pregnancy. ART includes procedures such as *in vitro fertilization (IVF)*, *gamete intra-fallopian transfer (GIFT)* and *zygote intra-fallopian transfer (ZIFT)*.

In *IVF*, ova (eggs) collected from the female reproductive tract are inseminated with sperm and allowed to fertilize in vitro. The resulting embryos are then transferred back to the patient. If the fertilized egg (or zygote stage) is transferred back, the term *ZIFT* is used.

If the ova and sperm are transferred to the anterior of the uterus before in vitro fertilization, the term *GIFT* is used.

If a sperm is injected into the egg instead of incubating ova with numerous sperm, then the process is called *intracytoplasmic sperm injection (ICSI)*.

When sperm are microsurgically aspirated from the epididymis for ICSI, the process is called *microscopic epididymal sperm aspiration (MESA)*. When sperm are non-surgically aspirated with a needle from the epididymis, the process is called *percutaneous epididymal sperm aspiration (PESA)*. However, when sperm are extracted directly from the testis, the process is called *testicular sperm extraction (TESE)*. Sperm aspirated with a needle from the testis is called *percutaneous testicular sperm extraction (PTSE)* or *testicular fine-needle aspiration (TFNA)*. For instances where no sperm cells are present, spermatids or spermatid nuclei can be removed directly from the testes for *round spermatid injection (ROSI)* or *round spermatid nuclear injection (ROSNI)* into the oocyte.

Suggested additional reading

Handbook of Andrology (1998). The American Society of Andrology. Lawrence, Allen Press.

Insler, V. & Lunenfeld, B. (eds.) (1993). *Infertility Male and Female.* Edinburgh: Churchill Livingstone.

Jeyendran, R. S. (1998). Semen analysis: method and interpretation. In *Gynecology and Obstetrics.* ed. J. J. Sciarra, vol. 5, ch. 64, pp. 1–15. Philadelphia: J. P. Lippincott Company.

Keel, B. A. & Webster, B. W. (eds.) (1990). *The Handbook of Laboratory Diagnosis and Treatment of Infertility.* Boca Raton: CRC Press.

Mortimer, D. (ed.) (1994). *Practical Laboratory Andrology.* New York: Oxford University Press.

Rowe, P. J., Comhaire, F. H., Hargreave, T. B. & Mellows, H. J. (eds.) (1993). *WHO Manual for the Standardized Investigation and Diagnosis of the Infertile Couple.* Cambridge: Cambridge University Press.

Rowe, P. J., Comhaire, F. H., Hargreave, T. B. & Mahmoud, A. M. A. (2000). *WHO Manual for the Standardized Investigation, Diagnosis and Management of the Infertile Male.* Cambridge: Cambridge University Press.

WHO Laboratory Manual for the Examination of Human Semen and Sperm–Cervical Mucus Interaction. (1999). World Health Organization, Cambridge, Cambridge University Press.

Zaneveld, L. J. D. & Jeyendran, R. S. (1992). Sperm function tests. In *Infertility and Reproductive Medicine Clinics of North America*, ed. J. W. Overstreet, pp. 353–71. Philadelphia: W. B. Saunders Company.

Zaneveld, L. J. D., Jeyendran, R. S., Vermeiden, J. P. W. & Lens, J. W. (1996). Sperm enzymes for diagnostic purposes. In *Human Spermatozoa in Assisted Reproduction*, ed. A. A. Acosta & T. F. Kruger, pp. 165–76. New York: The Pathenon Publisher Group.

Suggested additional reading

Index

chemotherapeutic agents 39
chlorambucil 39
chromatids, male 19
chromatin condensation 64
chromosomal abnormalities 38
chromosomes 3, 10
    haploid number in sperm nucleus
        64
chymotrypsin 24
citric acid 12, 22
cleavage spindle 19
coagulating proteins 12
coagulation 23–4, 79
coagulum *see* seminal coagulum
coitus
    interruptus 15, 33
    seminal pouch collection 15
colchicine 39, 41
collection of semen 15–16, 33
    container 48
    motility of sperm 47
colliculus seminalis obstruction 71
color of semen 24–5, 32
computer-aided sperm analysis (CASA)
        45
concentration of sperm 37–44
congenital factors 41
corona radiata 3, 19
corpus cavernosum 12
corpus spongiosum 12–13
Cowper's gland 11, 12
    fluid 14
creatine phosphokinase 68, 69
cryopreservation 1, 71
    membrane damage 59
cryptorchidism 40
cumulus oophorus 3, 19
cyclophosphamide 39
cystic fibrosis 38
cytokines 31
cytoplasmic droplet 17, 51–2

diabetes mellitus 40, 72
1,2-dibromochloropropane-117
        42
5a-dihydrotestosterone 13
diploidy 19
DNA 64
dyneins 48

ejaculate
    analysis 1, 15–16
    fertile 5–7
    fertilizing capacity 5
    infertile 7
    microorganisms 33–4
    transportation 16
    turbidity 23
    volume 38
ejaculation 13–14

ejaculatory ducts 11
    obstruction 24, 38, 71
electron microscopy 51
electro-stimulation 15
emission 13–14
endometrial cell cilia 18
epididymis 9, 11, 14, 79
    α-glucosidase production 70
    obstruction 38
    partial obstruction 40
epithelial cells 33
erythrocytes 32–3, 79
17β-estradiol 13
ethanol 42
ethylene dibromide 42
external urethral meatus 14

fallopian tubes
    ampullae 17, 18
    sperm transport 18
F–D method 65
female fertility
    analysis 1
    status 3
fertile sperm competency 7
fertility *see* female fertility; male fertility
fertilization 18–19
    antisperm antibodies 67
    site 17, 18
fever
    morphology of sperm 51–2
    motility of sperm 48
    see also infections
follicle-stimulating hormone (FSH) 13,
        39
free oxygen radicals 31, 48, 69
Friberg test 65
fructose 12, 22, 29, 30, 70–3, 79
    absence 38
furadantin 52

gelatin agglutination test 65
genetic mutation transmission ix–x,
        44
germ cells 10
    immature 32
    Klinefelter's syndrome 38
germinal cell aplasia 39
glans penis 12
glass wool 5–6, 7, 50
a-glucosidase 22, 38, 70–3, 79
glycoproteins 48
gonadotrophin-releasing hormone
        (GnRH) 13
guanethidine 30, 40, 72

heat *see* thermal stress
hematospermia 25, 32–3
hemizona binding test 61, 77, 78
hemocytometer counting chamber 37

chemical analysis 22, 70–5, 78, 87
clinical factors 72
count 79
pH 73–5, 78, 79
therapeutic factors 72
seminal pouch collection 15
seminal vesicles 11–12, 79
congenital absence 24, 38, 72
fructose production 70
obstruction 29
secretions 14
seminiferous tubules 10
diameter 38
Sephadex 5–6, 50
Sertoli cells 10, 13
germinal cell aplasia due to Sertoli
cells only 39
Klinefelter's syndrome 38
Sertoli cells only syndrome 39
sexual abstinence period 16
motility of sperm 47
oligozoospermia 40
sexual stimulation 15
motility of sperm 47
sexually transmissible disease 38
Shullman–Heckman method 65
signal transduction 69
silica colloidal suspension 5, 50
slide agglutination test 65
somatic nervous system 14
sperm(atozoa) 9
anatomy 16–17
antigenicity 65
aspiration 1
assays 2
biochemical analysis 22, 68–9, 78,
87
concentration 2, 89
count 37–44, 79
delivery path 38
fertility assay 82
fertility potential 2, 5
fertilizing capacity 69
immobilization test 65, 78
maturation 11, 67
migration time 18
physiology 17–18
quality 89
quality panel 77–8
removal 17, 50
selection techniques 5–6
storage 11
subfertile 6–7
surface binding 78
transport 11, 18, 47, 67
ultrastructural evaluation 78
washing through density gradients
5
see also morphology of sperm;
motility of sperm

sperm agglutination 31, 36, 78
infections 66
sperm function evaluation 2
sperm function tests 21–3, 55–63
hemizona binding test 61
panel 78
sperm acrosome reaction test 60
sperm membrane integrity test
58–9
sperm mucus penetration test 57
sperm nucleus integrity tests 64
sperm penetration test 62–3
sperm head 19, 68
fusion with oocyte vitelline
membrane 3
lateral movement 45
sperm membrane
alterations 77
integrity test 58–9
sperm mucus penetration test 57, 78
sperm nucleus 17
decondensation 3
integrity tests 22, 64
stability 64
sperm penetration test 62–3, 77, 78
sperm tail 19
amplitude 45
spermatids 34–5
cell wall 17
spermatocytes 10, 34–5
spermatogenesis 10, 13
antisperm antibodies 67
arrested 38
environmental pollutants 42
spermatogenic maturation arrest 39
spermatogonia 10, 34–5
spermiogenesis 10
sperm–oocyte contact 2–3
sperm–oocyte interaction 18–19
spinnbarkeit 25–6
spironolactone 41
stanozolol 40
stress factors 52
subfertility 6–7, 32
sulfasalazine 39, 41
superoxide anion 69
supravital test 58–9
surface-bound antibody 67
Swim-Up method 5, 50
sympathetic nervous system 14

teratozoospermia 51, 53, 54, 89
testis 9–11, 79
antibody production 39
testicular feminization 13
testicular sperm extraction (TESE) 1,
91
testosterone 13
thermal stress 40, 43, 52
thioridazine 30, 72

Printed in the United States
By Bookmasters